Essential Orthopedic Review

Adam E. M. Eltorai • Craig P. Eberson
Alan H. Daniels

Editors

Essential Orthopedic Review

Questions and Answers for Senior Medical Students

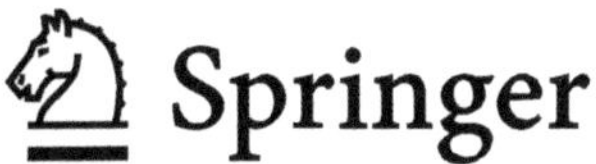 Springer

Editors
Adam E. M. Eltorai
Warren Alpert Medical School
Brown University
Providence, RI
USA

Alan H. Daniels
Department of Orthopedic
Surgery
Warren Alpert Medical School
Brown University
Providence, RI
USA

Craig P. Eberson
Department of Orthopedic
Surgery
Warren Alpert Medical School
Brown University
Providence, RI
USA

ISBN 978-3-319-78386-4   ISBN 978-3-319-78387-1   (eBook)
https://doi.org/10.1007/978-3-319-78387-1

Library of Congress Control Number: 2018943261

This Springer imprint is published by the registered company Springer International Publishing AG part of Springer Nature
The registered company address is: Gewerbestrasse 11, 6330 Cham, Switzerland

*This book is dedicated to
my wonderfully supportive
wife Michelle and my
children Theodore and
Anne, the loves of my life.*
Alan H. Daniels

*To Denise and my boys,
who make everything
worthwhile.*
Craig P. Eberson

For Ashley, always.
Adam E. M. Eltorai

Preface

The book is the ideal, on-the-spot reference for students seeking fast facts on diagnosis and management in orthopedic surgery.

Its two-column, question-and-answer format makes it a perfect quick reference. Organized by body part, *Essential Orthopedic Review* focuses on the most common pathologic entities. Topics include history, typical presentation, relevant anatomy, physical examination, imaging, management, and expected outcomes.

Essential Orthopedic Review is the ideal addition to a white coat pocket, allowing busy students to efficiently review fundamental principles in orthopedic surgery. Students can read specific chapters for focused subspecialty review or from cover to cover to lay a general foundation of orthopedic knowledge. Aimed at helping students start their orthopedic journeys on the right foot, this book will serve as a tool to propel students to the next level.

Providence, RI, USA

Adam E. M. Eltorai
Craig P. Eberson
Alan H. Daniels

Contents

Contributors

Laura Amorese-O'Connell, MD The Warren Alpert Medical School of Brown University, Providence, RI, USA

Jacob Babu, MD, MHA Department of Orthopaedic Surgery, Warren Alpert Medical School of Brown University, Rhode Island Hospital, Providence, RI, USA

Jason T. Bariteau, MD Department of Orthopaedic Surgery, Emory University School of Medicine, Atlanta, GA, USA

Brad D. Blankenhorn, MD Department of Orthopaedic Surgery, Warren Alpert Medical School of Brown University, Providence, RI, USA

Travis Blood, MD Department of Orthopaedics, Warren Alpert Medical School of Brown University, Providence, RI, USA

Alexandre Boulos, MD Department of Orthopaedics, Brown University, Providence, RI, USA

Tina Brar, MD Division of Rheumatology, The Warren Alpert School of Medicine of Brown University, Providence, RI, USA

Brian H. Cohen, MD Department of Orthopedic Surgery, Warren Alpert Medical School of Brown University, Providence, RI, USA

Aristides I. Cruz Jr., MD, MBA Department of Orthopaedic Surgery, Warren Alpert Medical School of Brown University, Providence, RI, USA

Joanne Szczygiel Cunha, **MD** Division of Rheumatology, The Warren Alpert School of Medicine of Brown University, Providence, RI, USA

Deepan Dalal, MD, MPH Department of Medicine-Rheumatology, Brown University, Providence, RI, USA

Manuel F. DaSilva, **MD** Department of Orthopedic Surgery, Warren Alpert Medical School of Brown University, Providence, RI, USA

Steven F. DeFroda, **MD, ME** Department of Orthopaedic Surgery, Warren Alpert Medical School of Brown University, Providence, RI, USA

Jeanne Delgado, **MD** Children's National Medical Center, Washington, DC, USA

Adam Driesman, MD Department of Orthopaedics, NYU Langone Orthopedic Hospital, New York, NY, USA

Drs. Ramirez and Terek are at associated with Brown University, Providence, RI, USA

Sean Esmende, **MD** Department of Orthopaedic Surgery, New England Musculoskeletal Institute, University of Connecticut School of Medicine, Farmington, CT, USA

Orthopedic Associates of Hartford, Division of Spine Surgery, The Bone and Joint Institute, Hartford Hospital, Hartford, CT, USA

Ross Feller, **MD** The Warren Alpert Medical School of Brown University, Providence, RI, USA

Avi DeLano Goodman, **MD** Department of Orthopaedics, Warren Alpert Medical School of Brown University, Providence, RI, USA

Heather Hansen, **MD** Division of Pediatric Orthopaedic Surgery, Department of Orthopaedics, The Warren Alpert Medical School of Brown University, Providence, RI, USA

Andrew Paul Harris, MD Department of Orthopedic Surgery, Warren Alpert Medical School of Brown University, Providence, RI, USA

Jonathan Hodax, **MD, MS** Department of Orthopedics, Rhode Island Hospital, Providence, RI, USA

Rishin J. Kadakia, **MD** Department of Orthopaedic Surgery, Emory University School of Medicine, Atlanta, GA, USA

Dominic Kleinhenz, **MD** Rhode Island Hospital Orthopaedic Surgery Residency Program, Brown University of Warren Alpert School of Medicine, Providence, RI, USA

Eren O. Kuris, **MD** Department of Orthopaedic Surgery, Warren Alpert Medical School of Brown University, Providence, RI, USA

Nicholas Lemme, **MD** Department of Orthopedics, Brown University, Providence, RI, USA

James Levins, **MD** Department of Orthopaedic Surgery, Brown University, Providence, RI, USA

Pieusha Malhotra, **MD, MPH** Department of Medicine-Rheumatology, Roger Williams Medical Center, Providence, RI, USA

P. Kaveh Mansuripur, **MD** Hand and Upper Limb Surgery, Stanford University School of Medicine, Stanford, CA, USA

Stephen Marcaccio, **MD** Department of Orthopaedic Surgery, Rhode Island Hospital, Brown University, Providence, RI, USA

Christopher Nacca, **MD** Department of Orthopaedics, Warren Alpert School of Medicine at Brown University, Providence, RI, USA

Seth W. O'Donnell, **MD** Division of Pediatric Orthopaedic Surgery, Department of Orthopaedic Surgery, Warren Alpert Medical School of Brown University, Providence, RI, USA

Devan Patel, **MD** Department of Orthopaedic Surgery, Warren Alpert Medical School of Brown University, Providence, RI, USA

Janake Patel, MD Roger William Medical Center, Boston University, Boston, MA, USA

Tyler S. Pidgeon, **MD** Department of Orthopaedic Surgery, The Warren Alpert Medical School at Brown University, Providence, RI, USA

Viorel Raducan, **MD, FRCS(C)** Department of Orthopaedic Surgery, Marshall University School of Medicine, Huntington, WV, USA

Jeremy E. Raducha, **MD** Department of Orthopaedic Surgery, Warren Alpert Medical School of Brown University, Providence, RI, USA

Jose M. Ramirez, **MD** Department of Orthopaedic Surgery, Alpert Medical School of Brown University, Providence, RI, USA

Daniel Brian Carlin Reid, **MD, MPH** Department of Orthopaedics, Rhode Island Hospital, Brown University, Providence, RI, USA

Jonathan R. Schiller, **MD** Adolescent and Young Adult Hip Program, Orthopaedic Surgery, The Warren Alpert School of Medicine of Brown University, Providence, RI, USA

Division of Pediatric Orthopaedics and Scoliosis, Hasbro Children's Hospital, Rhode Island Hospital, Providence, RI, USA

Division of Sports Medicine, Hasbro Children's Hospital, Rhode Island Hospital, Providence, RI, USA

Stuart T. Schwartz, **MD** Alpert Medical School of Brown University, Providence, RI, USA

Kalpit N. Shah, MD Department of Orthopaedic Surgery, Warren Alpert School of Medicine at Brown University, Providence, RI, USA

Hardeep Singh, **MD** Department of Orthopaedic Surgery, New England Musculoskeletal Institute, University of Connecticut School of Medicine, Farmington, CT, USA

Andrew D. Sobel, MD Department of Orthopedics, Warren Alpert Medical School of Brown University, Providence, RI, USA

Richard Terek, MD Warren Alpert Medical School of Brown University, Providence, RI, USA

John R. Tuttle, **MD, MS** Sports Medicine, Department of Orthopaedic Surgery, Virginia Tech Carilion School of Medicine, Roanoke, VA, USA

Gregory R. Waryasz, **MD, CSCS** Department of Orthopaedic Surgery, Massachusetts General Hospital, Boston, MA, USA

Part I
The Basics

Chapter 1
Orthopaedic Terminology

Jeremy E. Raducha

What do the following abbreviations stand for?	ORIF? A: Open reduction and internal fixation
	CRPP? A: Closed reduction and percutaneous pinning
	WBAT? A: Weight bearing as tolerated
	NWB? A: Non weight bearing
	FROM? A: Full range of motion
	THA? A: Total hip arthroplasty
	TKA? A: Total knee arthroplasty

(continued)

American Academy of Orthopaedic Surgery. AAOS—OrthoInfo: Glossary. American Academy of Orthopaedic Surgery webpage. http://orthoinfo.aaos.org/glossary.cfm. Published 2017. Accessed 24 Apr 2017.

J. E. Raducha, MD
Department of Orthopaedic Surgery, Warren Alpert Medical School, Brown University, Providence, RI, USA

© Springer International Publishing AG, part of Springer Nature 2018
A. E. M. Eltorai et al. (eds.), *Essential Orthopedic Review*,
https://doi.org/10.1007/978-3-319-78387-1_1

(continued)

What is an open fracture?	Fracture with communication between the bone and outside of the skin
What is the difference between a ligament and a tendon?	Ligament connects bone to bone, tendon connects muscle to bone
What is an external fixator?	Device positioned with pins into the two ends of a fractured bone or dislocation with bars outside of the skin. It is used to immobilize bones and joints. Most commonly used while waiting for soft tissues to become appropriate for internal fixation
Define arthroplasty	Reconstructive surgery of a joint (i.e. joint replacement)
Define arthrodesis	Surgical fusion of a joint
Define arthrocentesis	Removal of fluid from a joint
Define osteotomy	Surgical procedure that changes the alignment of bone
Define arthroscopy	Surgical procedure to diagnose and treat problems inside a joint using a minimally invasive scope
Define sprain	Partial or complete tear of a ligament
Define strain	Partial or complete tear of a muscle or tendon
Define varus	Distal segment angled toward anatomic midline
Define valgus	Distal segment angled away from anatomic midline

Chapter 2
Radiology: The Basics

Hardeep Singh and Sean Esmende

What is a systematic approach in reading an X-ray?	ABCS A: Adequacy and alignment B: Bones C: Cartilage (including joint spaces) S: Soft Tissues (effusions and swelling)
What is the appropriate initial study to obtain when suspecting a fracture?	Plain X-rays in orthogonal planes of the affected extremity

(continued)

H. Singh, MD
Department of Orthopaedic Surgery, New England
Musculoskeletal Institute, University of Connecticut School
of Medicine, Farmington, CT, USA
e-mail: hasingh@uchc.edu

S. Esmende, MD (✉)
Orthopedic Associates of Hartford, Division of Spine Surgery,
The Bone and Joint Institute, Hartford Hospital,
Hartford, CT, USA

© Springer International Publishing AG, part of Springer Nature 2018   5
A. E. M. Eltorai et al. (eds.), *Essential Orthopedic Review*,
https://doi.org/10.1007/978-3-319-78387-1_2

(continued)

What is the study of choice when suspicious of a stress fracture?	Magnetic resonance imaging (MRI) of the affected extremity
What is an important study to obtain when evaluating a fracture with intraarticular extension?	Computed tomography (CT) of the affected extremity for surgical planning
Which imaging study allows for assessment of soft tissue, ligaments, and tendons?	Magnetic resonance imaging (MRI)
Which are the five radiographic densities?	Air, Fat, Soft tissue/Fluid, Mineral, and Metal
What are the advantages of a CT scan over X-rays?	Allows for multiplanar visualization with the ability to reconstruct images to examine fine bony anatomy
How is a fracture identified on an X-ray?	Disruption (complete or incomplete) in the cortex of a bone
How are displacement, angulation, shortening, and rotation described on imaging studies?	With respect to the relationship of the distal fragment to the proximal fragment

Chapter 3
Fractures

Jeremy E. Raducha

<table>
<tr>
<td>

What pattern
of fracture is
demonstrated
in images A–E?

</td>
<td>

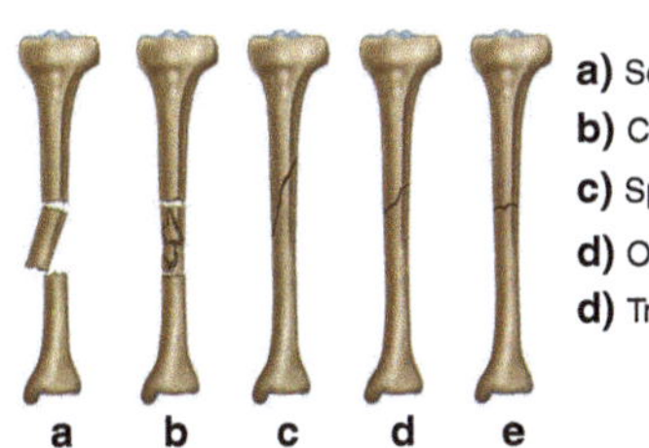

</td>
</tr>
<tr>
<td>

What fracture segment
is used to determine the
direction of angulation?

</td>
<td>

Distal segment

</td>
</tr>
</table>

(continued)

J. E. Raducha, MD
Department of Orthopaedic Surgery, Warren Alpert Medical
School of Brown University, Providence, RI, USA

© Springer International Publishing AG, part of Springer Nature 2018   7
A. E. M. Eltorai et al. (eds.), *Essential Orthopedic Review*,
https://doi.org/10.1007/978-3-319-78387-1_3

(continued)

Define pathological fracture	Fracture through abnormal bone (e.g. osteoporosis, tumour)
Define non-union	Failure of fractured bone pieces to fuse together after typically sufficient healing time
What are the main types of non-union?	Hypertrophic, oligotrophic, and atrophic
Define malunion	Fusion of fractured bone pieces in inappropriate alignment
Define delayed union	Longer than expected duration for fusion of fractured bone pieces
What system is used to classify open fractures?	Gustilo and Anderson grading system
What type of antibiotic is given for a Grade I or II open fracture?	First-generation cephalosporin (e.g. cefazolin)
How long does the average bone take to heal?	6–8 weeks
Which type of bone heals faster, cortical or cancellous?	Cancellous

Chapter 4
Dislocations

Jacob Babu

What is a feared long-term complication of any joint dislocation?	Post-traumatic arthritis
What is the most frequently dislocated joint in the body?	Shoulder
What type of upper extremity dislocation is commonly missed and should be kept in mind?	Posterior shoulder dislocation
What is one of the biggest concerns of shoulder dislocation in the young vs. elderly patient population?	Recurrent instability (young) vs. rotator cuff tears (elderly)

(continued)

J. Babu, MD, MHA
Department of Orthopaedic Surgery, Warren Alpert Medical School of Brown University, Rhode Island Hospital, Providence, RI, USA
e-mail: jacob_babu@brown.edu

© Springer International Publishing AG, part of Springer Nature 2018   9
A. E. M. Eltorai et al. (eds.), *Essential Orthopedic Review*,
https://doi.org/10.1007/978-3-319-78387-1_4

(continued)

What structures are injured in volar and dorsal dislocation of the hand PIP joint, respectively?	Central slip and volar plate
What are the important physical exam findings suggestive of direction of hip dislocation?	Internal rotation(posterior dislocation) vs. external rotation(anterior dislocation) of the leg accompanied by extremity shortening
What is a major potential complication of a hip dislocation?	Avascular necrosis (AVN) of the femoral head
What is the appropriate initial management for a suspected knee dislocation with asymmetric pedal pulses?	Immediate attempted reduction via direct axial traction
What is the structure most likely to block reduction of a lateral subtalar dislocation?	Posterior tibial tendon

Chapter 5
Orthopedic Emergencies

Jacob Babu

What should be urgently done if skin-tenting overlying a fracture is noticed?	Open reduction if closed reduction is not successful in relieving skin pressure
What are two of the most important factors determining outcome after an open fracture?	Time to antibiotics and transfer to Level 1 Trauma Center
What is the classification system commonly utilized to describe open fractures?	Gustilo–Anderson classification
What should be done next if diminished pulses are appreciated in a traumatic lower extremity injury?	Ankle Brachial Index

(continued)

J. Babu, MD, MHA
Department of Orthopaedic Surgery, Warren Alpert Medical School of Brown University, Rhode Island Hospital, Providence, RI, USA
e-mail: jacob_babu@brown.edu

© Springer International Publishing AG, part of Springer Nature 2018
A. E. M. Eltorai et al. (eds.), *Essential Orthopedic Review*,
https://doi.org/10.1007/978-3-319-78387-1_5

(continued)

What physical exam findings can be suggestive of compartment syndrome?	Pain, pallor, paresthesias, pulselessness, paralysis
What diagnostic test can help practitioners identify compartment syndrome?	Compartment pressure measurements compared to diastolic blood pressure. DBP−CP <30 is indicative of compartment syndrome
What cell count from a joint aspiration can be suggestive of a septic joint?	Nucleated cell counts greater than 50–80,000
What is a major consequence of a missed septic joint?	Articular cartilage destruction from bacterial toxins and inflammatory cell enzymes
What utility can be obtained from performing an MRI prior to reduction of a cervical facet dislocation?	Identifying a disc herniation and optimal approach for stabilization of fracture/dislocation
What are some of the red flag symptoms of a lumbar disc herniation which may indicate cauda equina syndrome?	Bowel/bladder incontinence or retention, saddle anesthesia, progressive extremity weakness and numbness

Chapter 6
Principles of Trauma

Jacob Babu

What class of shock and what percentage of total body blood loss are indicated by normal blood pressure with an elevated heart rate?	Class II Shock and loss of 15–30% blood volume
Transfusion of what blood products are indicated in a 1:1:1 ratio?	Red blood cells, platelets, plasma
What serum marker value is indicative of adequate resuscitation?	Serum lactate levels <2 mmol/L
How much blood can be lost into the thigh from a single femur fracture?	1–2 L

(continued)

J. Babu, MD, MHA
Department of Orthopaedic Surgery, Warren Alpert Medical School of Brown University, Rhode Island Hospital, Providence, RI, USA
e-mail: jacob_babu@brown.edu

© Springer International Publishing AG, part of Springer Nature 2018   13
A. E. M. Eltorai et al. (eds.), *Essential Orthopedic Review*,
https://doi.org/10.1007/978-3-319-78387-1_6

(continued)

What Injury Severity Score (ISS) is considered a major trauma with >10% mortality?	An ISS of 15. ISS = sum of the squares of the three highest Abbreviated Injury Scores (AIS)
What should be done if pelvic instability is identified by exam and radiograph and the patient is hemodynamically unstable?	Placement of pelvic binder or clamped bedsheet centered around patient's greater trochanters
What X-ray views can help better identify pelvic ring fractures?	Inlet and outlet views
What are the options of damage control orthopedics management of a long bone fracture?	External fixation and skeletal traction
What radiographic finding is indicative of a scapulothoracic dissociation?	Displacement of the edge of scapula from the spinous process by >1 cm from the contralateral side
Is lower extremity trauma an indication for internal fixation of an otherwise uncomplicated humeral shaft fracture?	Yes

Part II
The Upper Extremity

Chapter 7
Upper Extremity Physical Exam

Tyler S. Pidgeon

What structure is likely affected in a patient with a positive fovea sign?	The Triangular Fibrocartilage Complex (TFCC)
Allen's test evaluates the connection of which two arteries with the palmar arches of the hand?	The ulnar artery and the radial artery
A positive Obrien's test is suspicious for an injury to what shoulder structure?	The glenoid labrum
A patient with an abnormal hook test at the elbow would be most likely to have weakness with what motion of the forearm?	Supination
Finkelstein's test evaluates patients for what wrist condition?	De Quervain's tenosynovitis (tenosynovitis of the first dorsal compartment of the wrist)

(continued)

T. S. Pidgeon, MD
Department of Orthopaedic Surgery, The Warren Alpert Medical School at Brown University, Providence, RI, USA

© Springer International Publishing AG, part of Springer Nature 2018   17
A. E. M. Eltorai et al. (eds.), *Essential Orthopedic Review*,
https://doi.org/10.1007/978-3-319-78387-1_7

(continued)

What is the most sensitive physical exam special test for the diagnosis of carpal tunnel syndrome?	Durkan's carpal compression test
A patient with pain during resisted wrist extension with an extended elbow is most likely to have what condition?	Lateral epicondylitis
Describe the performance and findings of apprehension testing in a patient with suspected shoulder instability	The patient is supine on the examination table to stabilize the scapula. The shoulder is passively externally rotated by the examiner with the shoulder abducted and the elbow flexed to 90°. The patient complains of pain or apprehension that the shoulder will dislocate with increasing external rotation. Symptoms are improved when the examiner applies anterior to posterior pressure over the shoulder
Testing of thumb interphalangeal joint flexion strength and index finger distal interphalangeal joint strength examines the function of what nerve?	The anterior interosseous nerve (branch of the median nerve)
Positive Tinel's sign over the medial elbow is suggestive of what condition?	Cubital tunnel syndrome (ulnar nerve compression neuropathy)

Chapter 8
Rotator Cuff Pathology

Christopher Nacca

How many rotator cuff tendons exist?	Four
Name the rotator cuff tendons [1, 2].	Supraspinatus, infraspinatus, subscapularis, teres minor
What is the innervation of the Teres minor?	Axillary nerve
Where does the subscapularis insert?	Lesser tuberosity
Which side of the tendon do most tears occur?	Articular side
Name structures within the rotator interval.	Capsule, SGHL, coracohumeral ligament

(continued)

C. Nacca, MD
Department of Orthopaedics, Warren Alpert School of Medicine at Brown University, Providence, RI, USA

© Springer International Publishing AG, part of Springer Nature 2018   19
A. E. M. Eltorai et al. (eds.), *Essential Orthopedic Review*,
https://doi.org/10.1007/978-3-319-78387-1_8

(continued)

Majority of tears include which tendons?	Supraspinatus, infraspinatus
Which symptom is a poor indicator for nonoperative management?	Night pain
Hornblower's sign is often associated with which tendon tear?	Teres minor
What is the treatment for patients with massive rotator cuff tears and associated glenohumeral arthritis	Reverse total shoulder arthroplasty

References

1. Millett PJ, Warth RJ. Posterosuperior rotator cuff tears. J Am Acad Orthop Surg. 2014;22(8):521–34. https://doi.org/10.5435/JAAOS-22-08-521.
2. Murray J, Gross L. Optimizing the management of full-thickness rotator cuff tears. J Am Acad Orthop Surg. 2013;21(12):767–71. https://doi.org/10.5435/JAAOS-21-12-767.

Chapter 9
Adhesive Capsulitis

Christopher Nacca

Which structure in the shoulder is most often involved? [1]	Joint capsule
How many stages of progression are there?	Four
What is the most common presentation?	Pain of insidious onset over several months
Patients often complain having difficulty with which activities?	Sleeping on affected side, combing hair, or reaching behind back
Who are the most common demographic affected?	Women aged 40–60 years old
Which endocrine disorders are often implicated?	Diabetes and hypothyroidism
How is this condition best diagnosed?	Physical exam

(continued)

C. Nacca, MD
Department of Orthopaedics, Warren Alpert School of Medicine at Brown University, Providence, RI, USA

© Springer International Publishing AG, part of Springer Nature 2018   21
A. E. M. Eltorai et al. (eds.), *Essential Orthopedic Review*,
https://doi.org/10.1007/978-3-319-78387-1_9

(continued)

Which exam finding is most specific?	Limited passive range of motion in external rotation
What is the mainstay of treatment?	Intra-articular corticosteroid injection and physical therapy
How much time may it take for resolution of symptoms with nonoperative treatment?	Up to 2 years

References

1. Neviaser AS, Neviaser RJ. Adhesive capsulitis of the shoulder. J Am Acad Orthop Surg. 2011;19(9):536–42. http://www.ncbi.nlm. nih.gov/pubmed/21885699. Accessed 12 Jul 2017.

Chapter 10
Calcific Tendinitis

Kalpit N. Shah

What is calcific tendinitis?	Calcification and tendon deposition of the rotator cuff tendons at their insertion on the humerus
Who are the typical patients that develop calcific tendinitis?	Women aged 30–60 years
Which is the most common tendon involved?	Supraspinatus
Which medical comorbidities are risk factors?	Endocrine abnormalities—Hypothyroidism, diabetes
What are the three phases of calcific tendinitis?	Formative (calcium deposits being made) Resting (no inflammatory activity) Resorptive (phagocytic resorption—inflammatory mediators cause a significant amount of pain)

(continued)

K. N. Shah, MD
Department of Orthopaedic Surgery, Warren Alpert School of Medicine at Brown University, Providence, RI, USA

© Springer International Publishing AG, part of Springer Nature 2018   23
A. E. M. Eltorai et al. (eds.), *Essential Orthopedic Review*,
https://doi.org/10.1007/978-3-319-78387-1_10

(continued)

Which physical exam maneuvers are positive?	Subacromial impingement tests
What imaging modality is ideal?	Shoulder radiographs should show the calcium deposits at the insertion side of the various tendons
Where are the calcium deposits located?	1–1.5 cm away from the tendon insertion
What is the first-line treatment for calcific tendinitis?	Conservative: NSAIDs, therapy—stretching, strengthening, +/− steroid injections
What % of patients will improve with nonoperative management?	60–70% of patients by 6 months
What are the treatment options if patient fails conservative management?	Extracorporeal shockwave therapy Needle barbotage Surgical debridement

Chapter 11
Proximal Humeral Fracture

Avi DeLano Goodman

What X-ray views are needed?	Trauma series: true AP, axillary lateral, scapular Y
What defines a "part" in the Neer classification?	1 cm displacement or 45° angulation. Parts can be: greater tuberosity, lesser tuberosity, articular surface, and shaft
Which is the most common type of fracture?	Surgical neck (85%)
What is the incidence of nerve injury, and which nerve is most commonly injured?	45%, axillary nerve
What is the blood supply to the humeral head?	Anterior humeral circumflex artery (old data), posterior humeral circumflex artery (new data)

(continued)

A. D. Goodman, MD
Department of Orthopaedics, Warren Alpert Medical School
of Brown University, Providence, RI, USA
e-mail: avi_goodman@brown.edu

© Springer International Publishing AG, part of Springer Nature 2018
A. E. M. Eltorai et al. (eds.), *Essential Orthopedic Review*,
https://doi.org/10.1007/978-3-319-78387-1_11

(continued)

What is attached to each tuberosity?	Greater: rotator cuff (will displace superiorly and posteriorly) Lesser: subscapularis (will rotate internally)
When to consider nonoperative management?	Minimally displaced, greater tuberosity displacement <5 mm, low demand, otherwise not medically able to undergo surgery
What are the surgical options?	ORIF, intramedullary nail, CRPP, and arthroplasty (hemiarthroplasty, anatomic total, and reverse total)
What are the common complications?	Intraarticular screw penetration, avascular necrosis, malunion, nonunion, rotator cuff injury, posttraumatic arthritis, stiffness

Chapter 12
Clavicular Fracture

Jonathan Hodax

How is the clavicle formed in embryology and childhood development?	Intramembranous ossification
What is special about the clavicle's timing of ossification?	First bone to begin to ossify, last to finish
What side does congenital pseudoarthrosis of the clavicle typically occur on and why?	RIGHT side, believed to be because of the brachiocephalic artery
How are clavicle fractures typically grouped?	Medial, middle, and lateral third
How are medial clavicle fractures classified?	Anterior versus posterior displacement

(continued)

J. Hodax, MD, MS
Department of Orthopedics, Rhode Island Hospital, Providence, RI, USA

© Springer International Publishing AG, part of Springer Nature 2018   27
A. E. M. Eltorai et al. (eds.), *Essential Orthopedic Review*,
https://doi.org/10.1007/978-3-319-78387-1_12

(continued)

How are middle third clavicle fractures classified?	Typically displaced versus nondisplaced, comminuted versus not
How are lateral third clavicle fractures classified?	Neer classification, type I–V
What ligaments attach to the clavicle?	Costoclavicular ligament medially, and the conoid and trapezoid coracoclavicular ligaments laterally
What are the absolute indications to operate on a middle third clavicle fracture?	Open fracture, threatened skin, subclavian injury
What are the relative indications to operate on a middle third clavicle fracture?	Displacement greater than 100%, "Z" deformity, comminution, shortening more than 2 cm, polytrauma
What is the most common cause for reoperation after fixation of clavicle fractures?	Hardware removal

Chapter 13
AC Joint Separation

Jonathan Hodax

How are AC separations classified?	By the Rockwood classification
	I: Symptomatic sprain without radiographic displacement
	II: Coracoclavicular interval widening of up to 25% compared with contralateral III: Coracoclavicular interval widening of 25–100%
	IV: Clavicle displaced posteriorly into/through trapezius
	V: Clavicle displaced more than 100% superiorly, lateral end through deltotrapezial fascia
	VI: Inferiorly displaced lateral clavicle, with clavicle resting posterior to coracobrachialis tendon
What X-rays are best to evaluate AC joint injuries?	Zanca view and comparative images of the uninjured shoulder

(continued)

J. Hodax, MD, MS
Department of Orthopedics, Rhode Island Hospital, Providence, RI, USA

© Springer International Publishing AG, part of Springer Nature 2018
A. E. M. Eltorai et al. (eds.), *Essential Orthopedic Review*,
https://doi.org/10.1007/978-3-319-78387-1_13

(continued)

What AC separations are appropriate for surgical intervention?	Type IV and higher are generally operatively treated. Type III are operative in athletes or those who fail nonop treatment
What surgical techniques exist for repairing the AC joint?	Allograft reconstruction with tendon looped around the coranoid, screw fixation to the coranoid, and suture fixation of the clavicle to the coranoid
What portion of the AC joint capsule is strongest?	The posterosuperior joint capsule

Chapter 14
Glenohumeral Joint Pathology

Devan Patel

Is anterior or posterior instability more common?	Anterior
What is TUBS?	Traumatic unilateral shoulder dislocations, with a Bankart lesion often requiring surgery
What is AMBRI?	Atraumatic multidirectional bilateral shoulder dislocation often requiring rehabilitation and occasionally requiring inferior capsular shift
What is a Bankart lesion?	Disruption of the anterior inferior glenoid labrum, often a result of anterior shoulder dislocations
What is a Hill Sachs lesion?	Impaction injury to the posterior superior humeral head, often seen after an anterior dislocation

(continued)

D. Patel, MD
Department of Orthopaedic Surgery, Warren Alpert Medical School of Brown University, Providence, RI, USA
e-mail: Devan_Patel@brown.edu

© Springer International Publishing AG, part of Springer Nature 2018   31
A. E. M. Eltorai et al. (eds.), *Essential Orthopedic Review*,
https://doi.org/10.1007/978-3-319-78387-1_14

(continued)

What is the "lightbulb" sign?	Appearance of the humeral head in internal rotation on an AP radiograph seen after a posterior shoulder dislocation
What is a HAGL lesion?	Humeral avulsion of the inferior glenohumeral ligament, most commonly seen after an anterior shoulder dislocation
What incidents typically cause posterior dislocations?	High-energy trauma, seizures, and electrocution accidents
Which muscle group is the primary cause of posterior shoulder dislocations?	Shoulder internal rotators overpower external rotators
What portion of the glenoid typically appears most worn in osteoarthritis of the glenohumeral joint?	Posterior glenoid

Chapter 15
Upper Extremity Arthroplasty

Tyler S. Pidgeon

Total shoulder arthroplasty is contraindicated in patients with what soft-tissue shoulder pathology?	Rotator cuff deficiency (large and irreparable full-thickness tears/non-functional rotator cuff/ rotator cuff arthropathy)
What shoulder arthroplasty options are available to patients with rotator cuff deficiency?	Reverse total shoulder arthroplasty and shoulder hemiarthroplasty
Reverse total shoulder arthroplasty function relies on the function of what muscle?	Deltoid
Total shoulder arthroplasty in patients with rotator cuff deficiency fails most commonly by what mechanism?	Glenoid component loosening and failure

(continued)

T. S. Pidgeon, MD
Department of Orthopaedic Surgery, The Warren Alpert Medical School at Brown University, Providence, RI, USA

© Springer International Publishing AG, part of Springer Nature 2018
A. E. M. Eltorai et al. (eds.), *Essential Orthopedic Review*,
https://doi.org/10.1007/978-3-319-78387-1_15

(continued)

What indication for total elbow arthroplasty results in the longest survivorship?	Rheumatoid arthritis
What is the lifelong lifting restriction for patients who have undergone total elbow arthroplasty?	Repetitive activity: 2 pounds; Single lift activity: 5–10 pounds
The latest generation (fourth generation) total wrist arthroplasty designs have approximately what 5-year survival rate?	90–97%
Thumb carpal-metacarpal (CMC) joint arthroplasty most commonly involves resection of what carpal bone?	The trapezium
Attenuation of what ligament is thought to be a major contributing cause of thumb CMC arthritis?	The anterior oblique (Beak) ligament (primary stabilizer of the thumb CMC joint)
Silicon metacarpophalangeal (MCP) joint replacement of the index, middle, ring, and small finger during the same operation is most commonly performed for patients with what disease?	Rheumatoid arthritis

Chapter 16
Superior Labrum Anterior to Posterior Lesions

Jonathan Hodax

How are SLAP tears classified?	By the Tuoheti classification I: Fraying of the superior labrum with an intact biceps anchor II: Superior labral detachment with detachment of the biceps anchor III: Bucket-handle type tear of the superior labrum, biceps anchor intact IV: Bucket handle tear of the labrum with extension into the biceps tendon, anchor partially intact
How are SLAP tears typically treated?	Type I: Debride frayed edge Type II: Debride and reattach biceps and labrum Type III: Resect tear, anchor free edges if needed Type IV: Resect tear. If >50% of biceps tendon involved, consider tenodesis

(continued)

J. Hodax, MD, MS
Department of Orthopedics, Rhode Island Hospital, Providence, RI, USA

© Springer International Publishing AG, part of Springer Nature 2018   35
A. E. M. Eltorai et al. (eds.), *Essential Orthopedic Review*,
https://doi.org/10.1007/978-3-319-78387-1_16

(continued)

In what population are SLAP tears most clinically significant?	Overhead throwing athletes
What is a cordlike MGHL with absence of the anterior labrum called? And should this be repaired down?	A Buford complex, and NO!
What is the major surgical pitfall to avoid in SLAP repairs?	Overconstraint of the biceps tendon leading to reduced range of motion

Chapter 17
Biceps Tendon Ruptures

Kalpit N. Shah

Where do the two heads of the biceps tendon originate from?	Coracoid process (short head) and the superior glenoid (long head)
Where does the biceps tendon attach distally?	Bicipital tuberosity of the radius Long head attaches proximally Short head attaches distally
Where does the lacertus fibrosus originate and insert?	Comes off the medial side of the short head of the biceps tendon in the antecubital fossa Crosses the antecubital fossa and is continuous with the deep fascia of the flexor muscle bellies
What innervate the biceps muscle?	Musculocutaneous nerve

(continued)

K. N. Shah, MD
Department of Orthopaedic Surgery, Warren Alpert School of Medicine at Brown University, Providence, RI, USA

© Springer International Publishing AG, part of Springer Nature 2018   37
A. E. M. Eltorai et al. (eds.), *Essential Orthopedic Review*,
https://doi.org/10.1007/978-3-319-78387-1_17

(continued)

What type of contraction leads to tendon injury?	Eccentric contraction—forced elbow extension when flexed
Can patients with biceps tendon rupture flex their elbow?	Yes, brachialis muscle is the primary elbow flexor. Biceps brachii contributes 30% of elbow flexion strength
Can patients with biceps tendon ruptures supinate their arm?	Yes, supinator contributes to forearm supination. Biceps brachii contributes roughly 40–50% of the supination strength
Physical exam test to assess distal biceps tendon?	Hook test—examiner tries to hook their index finger into the patient's biceps tendon in the antecubital fossa
If a patient has a known distal biceps tear, but still has a negative hook test, what structure is the examiner palpating?	Lacertus fibrosus
What deformity does a patient with a biceps rupture have on examination?	Popeye deformity
Best imaging test to evaluate for this injury?	MRI with the forearm flexed, supinated, and shoulder abducted
What nerve is at risk of being injured during surgical repair of distal biceps tendon?	Posterior interosseous nerve and lateral antebrachial cutaneous nerve

Chapter 18
Humeral Shaft Fracture

Devan Patel

How can humeral shaft fracture patterns be described?	Transverse, oblique, spiral, comminuted with or without butterfly fragments
What are the primary deforming forces of humeral shaft fractures?	Pectoralis major: adducts proximal fracture fragments Deltoid: abducts proximal fracture fragments
What are the maximum acceptable reduction criteria for nonoperative management?	Malrotation: 15° Anterior angulation: 20° Varus: 30° Shortening/bayonet opposition: 3 cm

(continued)

D. Patel, MD
Department of Orthopaedic Surgery, Warren Alpert Medical School of Brown University, Providence, RI, USA
e-mail: Devan_Patel@brown.edu

© Springer International Publishing AG, part of Springer Nature 2018   39
A. E. M. Eltorai et al. (eds.), *Essential Orthopedic Review*,
https://doi.org/10.1007/978-3-319-78387-1_18

(continued)

What is the classic mechanism of humeral shaft fractures?	High energy trauma → direct force → transverse and comminuted fractures Indirect trauma (fall on outstretched hand) → rotational forces → spiral fracture patterns
What are some associated neurovascular injuries with humeral shaft fractures?	Radial nerve injuries, brachial plexus injuries, and profunda brachii arteries
What are the indications for operative management?	Open fractures, unacceptable reduction criteria, radial nerve palsy after reduction, ipsilateral upper extremity injuries, pathological fractures, and segmental fractures
What is the most common nonoperative treatment?	Coaptation splint followed by Sarmiento brace or casting
What are the operative treatments for humeral shaft fractures?	Intramedullary nail, plate fixation, and external fixation
Common complications of a humeral shaft fracture include?	Radial nerve palsy, malunion, delayed union, non-union

Chapter 19
Tennis and Golfer's Elbow (Epicondylitis)

Andrew D. Sobel

What is the most common muscle origin affected in tennis elbow (lateral epicondylitis)?	Extensor carpi radialis brevis (ECRB)
What is the histopathology of lateral epicondylitis?	Angiofibroblastic hyperplasia and disorganized collagen
What are the two most common findings on examination of lateral epicondylitis?	Tenderness to palpation at lateral epicondyle/insertion of ECRB Pain with wrist extension against resistance
What is a common non-traumatic condition that can often be confused with lateral epicondylitis and how can you differentiate them on exam?	Radial tunnel syndrome which has pain more distal (3–4 cm) from the lateral epicondyle and pain with extension of the long finger

(continued)

A. D. Sobel, MD
Department of Orthopedics, Warren Alpert Medical School of Brown University, Providence, RI, USA

© Springer International Publishing AG, part of Springer Nature 2018   41
A. E. M. Eltorai et al. (eds.), *Essential Orthopedic Review*,
https://doi.org/10.1007/978-3-319-78387-1_19

(continued)

What is the most effective treatment for lateral epicondylitis?	Nonoperative with grip training (gripping/lifting with forearm supinated instead of pronated), physical therapy, corticosteroid injections, etc.
What is the cause of golfer's elbow (medial epicondylitis)?	Repetitive eccentric loading of flexor-pronator mass usually affecting all muscles except the palmaris longus
What neurologic disorder is often concomitantly present with medial epicondylitis?	Ulnar nerve compression/neuritis
What are classic exam findings for medial epicondylitis?	Tenderness to palpation 5–10 mm distal and anterior to the medial epicondyle and pain/weakness with resisted wrist flexion, forearm pronation, or grip
What is the most effective treatment for medial epicondylitis?	Nonoperative with counterforce bracing/taping, flexor-pronator mass stretching/strengthening. Corticosteroid injections should not be repeated multiple times

Chapter 20
Olecranon Bursitis

Travis Blood

What blood tests should be obtained with suspected infectious olecranon bursitis?	CBC with differential, ESR, CRP
What can you do to test the fluid of the bursa?	Sterile aspiration
What should you send the aspiration for?	Gram stain and culture
What is the most likely organism that is isolated from infected elbow bursitis?	Staphylococcal aureus
What nerve is on the medial side of the olecranon?	Ulnar nerve
Is elbow bursitis usually painful or non-painful?	Non-painful

T. Blood, MD
Department of Orthopaedics, Warren Alpert Medical School of
Brown University, Providence, RI, USA
e-mail: travis_blood@brown.edu

© Springer International Publishing AG, part of Springer Nature 2018   43
A. E. M. Eltorai et al. (eds.), *Essential Orthopedic Review*,
https://doi.org/10.1007/978-3-319-78387-1_20

Chapter 21
Distal Humerus Fractures

Devan Patel

What is the general classification of distal humerus fractures?	OTA/AO A—Extra-artricular (supracondylar) B—Partial articular (single column) C—Complete articular (bicolumn)
What is the classification system for partial articular single column fractures?	The Milch classification system I: Lateral trochlear ridge intact II: Fracture through the lateral trochlear ridge
What is the classification system for complete articular bicolumn fractures?	The Jupiter classification system
What imaging modality is important to better define these fracture patterns?	Computed tomography (CT) scanning

(continued)

D. Patel, MD
Department of Orthopaedic Surgery, Warren Alpert Medical School of Brown University, Providence, RI, USA
e-mail: Devan_Patel@brown.edu

© Springer International Publishing AG, part of Springer Nature 2018   45
A. E. M. Eltorai et al. (eds.), *Essential Orthopedic Review*,
https://doi.org/10.1007/978-3-319-78387-1_21

(continued)

What is the "double arch" sign?	Seen on lateral radiographs in coronal sheer fractures of the capitellum.
When is nonoperative management the treatment of choice?	Nondisplaced fractures, patients who are not surgical candidates due to other medical comorbidities, and advanced dementia
What is the "bag of bones" technique?	Nonoperative treatment of distal humerus fractures in a sling, used in patients with severe medical comorbidities
What are some operative options?	Closed reduction with percutaneous pinning, open reduction internal, distal humeral replacement, and total elbow arthroplasty
What are the surgical approaches to the elbow?	Triceps splitting, triceps sparing, triceps reflecting, and olecranon osteotomy
What are some common complications?	Stiffness, heterotopic ossification, ulnar nerve palsy, nonunion, and malunion

Chapter 22
Olecranon Fracture

Travis Blood

What tendon attaches to the posterior olecranon?	Triceps tendon
What is the most common treatment option for a simple transverse olecranon fracture?	Tension-band wiring
What articulates with the greater sigmoid notch of the ulna to form one of the elbow joints?	Trochlea of the distal humerus
What is the purpose of the olecranon fossa of the elbow?	Increase extension arc of motion and decrease impingement

(continued)

T. Blood, MD
Department of Orthopaedics, Warren Alpert Medical School
of Brown University, Providence, RI, USA
e-mail: travis_blood@brown.edu

© Springer International Publishing AG, part of Springer Nature 2018   47
A. E. M. Eltorai et al. (eds.), *Essential Orthopedic Review*,
https://doi.org/10.1007/978-3-319-78387-1_22

(continued)

If there is an olecranon fracture and dislocation of the radius what direction will the radius most likely dislocate?	Anteriorly
What are the treatment options for displaced olecranon fractures?	Tension band wiring, plate and screw fixation, intramedullary rod, excision and triceps advancement
What is the number one reason for return to operating room after fixation of olecranon fracture?	Removal of hardware, hardware irritation

Chapter 23
Radial Head Fractures

Kalpit N. Shah

What position of the arm during a fall causes a radial fracture?	Elbow fully extended and forearm pronated
What is the terrible triad of the elbow?	Elbow dislocation, radial head fracture, and coronoid fracture
What is an Essex-Lopresti injury?	Radial head fracture, interosseous membrane disruption, DRUJ injury
Most common classification for radial head fractures?	Mason classification Type I: Nondisplaced Type II: Displaced (>2 mm) with rotation block Type III: Comminuted and displaced Type IV: Elbow dislocation + radial head fracture

(continued)

K. N. Shah, MD
Department of Orthopaedic Surgery, Warren Alpert School of Medicine at Brown University, Providence, RI, USA

© Springer International Publishing AG, part of Springer Nature 2018   49
A. E. M. Eltorai et al. (eds.), *Essential Orthopedic Review*,
https://doi.org/10.1007/978-3-319-78387-1_23

(continued)

How to assess a block to forearm rotation in the setting of a radial head fracture?	Aspirate elbow hematoma and inject lidocaine (reduces pain associated with the fracture)
What is important if managing a nondisplaced radial head nonoperatively?	Early ROM (after few days in a sling) to avoid elbow stiffness
Surgical treatment options for radial head fractures?	ORIF, partial excision, full excision, radial head replacement
Fragments under what size should be excised?	Fragments<25% radial head articular surface should be excised
How to decide between fragment excision vs. radial head replacement?	Replace the radial head if more than three fragments need to be excised
Which nerve is at risk during a surgical approach to the radial head?	PIN—Avoid damaging this nerve with pronation of the forearm
What are safe zones for ORIF of radial head?	90° arc on the radial head that is in line with the radial styloid to the bicipital tuberosity

Chapter 24
Coranoid Fracture

Steven F. DeFroda

What injury is most associated with coranoid fracture?	Elbow dislocation
What important anatomic structure attaches just distal to the coranoid tip?	Anterior capsule of the elbow
What is a "terrible triad" injury?	Coranoid fracture, elbow dislocation, radial head fracture
Define the Regan and Morrey classification	Type 1: Coranoid tip Type 2: <50% of coranoid Type 3: >50% of coranoid
Is the coranoid an intra- or extra-articular structure?	Intra-articular
Where does the medial ulnar collateral ligament insert?	Medial facet

S. F. DeFroda, MD, ME
Department of Orthopaedic Surgery, Warren Alpert Medical School of Brown University, Providence, RI, USA

© Springer International Publishing AG, part of Springer Nature 2018   51
A. E. M. Eltorai et al. (eds.), *Essential Orthopedic Review*,
https://doi.org/10.1007/978-3-319-78387-1_24

References

1. Chen NC, Ring D. Terrible triad injuries of the elbow. J Hand Surg Am. 2015;40(11):2297–303. https://doi.org/10.1016/j.jhsa.2015.04.039.

Chapter 25
Elbow Dislocations

Devan Patel

How are elbow dislocation discribed in terms of direction?	The olecranon (distal) compared to the humerus (proximal)
What is the most common type of elbow dislocation?	Posterolateral
What are the primary static stabilizers of the elbow?	Joint capsule, anterior bundle of the medial collateral ligament, lateral collateral ligament complex, joint congruity
What are the dynamic stabilizers of the elbow?	Anconeus, brachailis, and triceps
In what direction do the stabilizing elements of the elbow fail during a dislocation?	Lateral to medial, from the LCL to the MCL

(continued)

D. Patel, MD
Department of Orthopaedic Surgery, Warren Alpert Medical School of Brown University, Providence, RI, USA
e-mail: Devan_Patel@brown.edu

© Springer International Publishing AG, part of Springer Nature 2018   53
A. E. M. Eltorai et al. (eds.), *Essential Orthopedic Review*,
https://doi.org/10.1007/978-3-319-78387-1_25

(continued)

What are surgical indications for an elbow dislocation?	Open injuries, gross instability of the elbow, and other elbow fractures that warrant operative intervention
What is the typical position of splinting elbow dislocations?	90° of flexion with forearm pronation
What is the terrible triad?	Elbow dislocation with a radial head and coronoid fracture
What are the complications of elbow dislocations?	Stiffness, pain, and instability

Chapter 26
Degenerative Joint Disease of the Elbow

Jeremy E. Raducha

What type of collagen is found most commonly in articular cartilage?	Type II collagen
What are the three articulations of the elbow?	Ulnotrochlear, radiocapitellar, and proximal radioulnar joints
What is the most common cause of elbow arthritis?	Rheumatoid arthritis

(continued)

Sanchez-Sotelo J, Morrey BF. Total elbow arthroplasty. J Am Acad Orthop Surg. 2011;19(2):121–5. http://www.ncbi.nlm.nih.gov/pubmed/21292935. Accessed 24 Apr 2017.

Kokkalis ZT, Schmidt CC, Sotereanos DG. Elbow arthritis: current concepts. J Hand Surg Am. 2009;34(4):761–8. doi:10.1016/j.jhsa.2009.02.019. Soojan MG, Kwon YW. Elbow arthritis. Bull NYU Hosp Jt Dis. 2007;65(1):61–71. http://presentationgrafix.com/_dev/cake/files/archive/pdfs/526.pdf. Accessed 26 Apr 2017.

J. E. Raducha, MD
Department of Orthopaedic Surgery, Warren Alpert Medical School of Brown University, Providence, RI, USA

© Springer International Publishing AG, part of Springer Nature 2018   55
A. E. M. Eltorai et al. (eds.), *Essential Orthopedic Review*,
https://doi.org/10.1007/978-3-319-78387-1_26

(continued)

Which motion is typically lost first in elbow arthritis?	Terminal extension
Which nerve is most likely affected by end stage elbow arthritis?	Ulnar nerve
Which indication for total elbow arthroplasty has the highest survivorship?	Rheumatoid arthritis
What are the absolute contraindications for total elbow arthroplasty?	Active infection and charcot joint
What is the most common complication following total elbow arthroplasty?	Infection

Chapter 27
Osteoarthritis of the Upper Extremity

Devan Patel

What are the symptoms of osteoarthritis?	Joint pain, swelling, decreased range of motion, and tenderness
What are the radiographic findings of osteoarthritis?	Osteophyte formation, sclerosis, joint space narrowing, and subchondral cysts
What are Heberden nodes?	Palpable osteophytes of the distal interphalangeal joint in the finger
Why is osteoarthritis in the DIP joints so common?	Increased force through this joint relative to others in the hand
What are Bouchard's nodes?	Palpable osteophytes of the proximal interphalangeal joint in the finger may occur due to osteoarthritis or rheumatoid arthritis

(continued)

D. Patel, MD
Department of Orthopaedic Surgery, Warren Alpert Medical School of Brown University, Providence, RI, USA
e-mail: Devan_Patel@brown.edu

© Springer International Publishing AG, part of Springer Nature 2018   57
A. E. M. Eltorai et al. (eds.), *Essential Orthopedic Review*,
https://doi.org/10.1007/978-3-319-78387-1_27

(continued)

Laxity in what ligament is thought to contribute to thumb CMC arthritis?	Anterior oblique ligament (beak ligament)
What are some physical exam findings seen in CMC arthritis?	Positive CMC grind test, "Z deformity," and adduction deformity
What are some conservative treatments to CMC arthritis?	Activity modification, NSADIS, steroid injections, and braces
What are surgical treatment options for CMC arthritis?	Trapezium resection, ligament reconstruction with or without tendon interposition, osteotomy, and arthrodesis

Chapter 28
Posttraumatic Arthritis: Elbow

Manuel F. DaSilva

What is the physiologic ROM of the elbow?	0–146 extension/flexion; 71° of forearm pronation and 84° of forearm supination
What is the elbow ROM required for most ADLs?	30–130° of flexion and extension
What is the best imaging modality to assess complex deformity?	3D reconstruction CT technology
How do you test for potential infection preoperatively?	Elbow aspiration for cell count with differential and cultures
What part of the medial collateral ligament (MCL) must be preserved during surgical release?	Anterior bundle of the MCL

(continued)

M. F. DaSilva, MD
Department of Orthopedic Surgery, Warren Alpert Medical School of Brown University, Providence, RI, USA
e-mail: Manuel_Dasilva@brown.edu

© Springer International Publishing AG, part of Springer Nature 2018
A. E. M. Eltorai et al. (eds.), *Essential Orthopedic Review*,
https://doi.org/10.1007/978-3-319-78387-1_28

(continued)

To increase flexion doing surgical release what part of the MCL ligament must be released?	Posterior bundle of the MCL
Define ulnohumeral arthroplasty.	Open or arthroscopic procedure that removes impinging osteophytes or loose bodies, synovectomy, and capsular release
What is the clinical presentation of patients with isolated radiocapitellar arthritis?	Lateral sided elbow pain with recurrent effusions
What is the common location for osteophytes that block motion?	Coronoid and olecranon fossae
What is the most common nerve complication of ulnohumeral arthroplasty?	Ulnar neuropathy
What are the restrictions for patients with total elbow arthroplasty?	10 lbs for single lift and under 2–5 lbs for repetitive lifting

Chapter 29
Radius and Ulnar Shaft Fractures

Jeremy E. Raducha

In addition to radius/ulna views which radiograph tests are required in patients with forearm fractures?	Ipsilateral elbow and wrist radiographs
What type of splint is used to initially immobilize radius/ulna diaphysis fractures?	Sugartong

(continued)

Baratz ME. Disorders of the forearm axis. In: Wolfe SWM, editor. Green's operative hand surgery. 7th ed. Philadelphia: Elsevier; 2017. p. 786–812. https://www-clinicalkey-com.revproxy.brown.edu/service/content/pdf/watermarked/3-s2.0-B9781455774272000216.pdf?locale=en_US. Accessed 18 Apr 2017.Gaulke R. Diaphyseal fractures of the forearm. In: Browner B, et al., editor. Skeletal trauma: basic science, management, and reconstruction. 5th ed. Philadelphia: Elsevier-Saunders; 2015. p. 1313–47. https://www-clinicalkey-com.revproxy.brown.edu/service/content/pdf/watermarked/3-s2.0-B9781455776283000454.pdf?locale=en_US. Accessed 23 Apr 2017.

J. E. Raducha, MD
Department of Orthopaedic Surgery, Warren Alpert Medical School of Brown University, Providence, RI, USA

© Springer International Publishing AG, part of Springer Nature 2018   61
A. E. M. Eltorai et al. (eds.), *Essential Orthopedic Review*,
https://doi.org/10.1007/978-3-319-78387-1_29

(continued)

What is a "both bone" fracture?	Fracture of both the radius and ulna at the same level
What is a "nightstick" fracture?	Isolated ulnar shaft fracture
What percent displacement is allowed for nonoperative treatment in a stable ulnar shaft fracture?	<50% displacement and <10° angulation
What is the most important variable in a functional outcome following radial and ulnar ORIF?	Restoration of the radial bow
What approaches are used for radial shaft ORIF?	Volar approach of Henry and dorsal (Thompson) approach
What are complications of radial/ulna ORIF?	Infection, synostosis, nonunion, malunion, compartment syndrome, neurovascular injury, re-fracture
What factor is associated with re-fracture of a surgically fixed radius/ulna fracture?	Premature plate removal, comminuted fracture, large plate, persistent lucency on X-ray

Chapter 30
Monteggia and Galeazzi Fracture/Dislocations

Devan Patel

What is a Monteggia fracture?	Proximal ulna fracture with a radial head dislocation
What is the common classification system for Monteggia fractures?	The Bado system Type I—Proximal/middle ulna fracture with an anterior radial head dislocation(most common) Type II—Proximal/middle ulna fracture with a posterior radial head dislocation Type III—Proximal/middle ulna fracture with a lateral radial head dislocation Type IV—Proximal/middle ulna and radius fracture with a radial head dislocation

(continued)

D. Patel, MD
Department of Orthopaedic Surgery, Warren Alpert Medical School of Brown University, Providence, RI, USA
e-mail: Devan_Patel@brown.edu

© Springer International Publishing AG, part of Springer Nature 2018   63
A. E. M. Eltorai et al. (eds.), *Essential Orthopedic Review*,
https://doi.org/10.1007/978-3-319-78387-1_30

(continued)

What nerve can be injured in patients with Monteggia fractures?	Posterior Interosseus Nerve (PIN) injury
What is the typical mechanism of injury in a Monteggia fracture?	Fall on outstretched arm in hyperpronation
What is a Galeazzi fracture?	Distal third radius fracture with a distal radial ulnar joint dislocation
What are some radiographic findings indicative of a DRUJ injury?	DRUJ widening greater than 5 mm Ulnar styloid fracture Radial shortening
What are the deforming forces in a Galeazzi fracture?	Brachioradialis → pulls distal fragment proximally Pronator quadratus → pronates the fragment and pulls it volarly
What is the typical treatment for Galeazzi fractures?	Operative to achieve, fixation of the radius and stabilization of the DRUJ
What is an Essex-Lopresti lesion?	A radial head fracture with an associated interosseus membrane and DRUJ disruption
What are key physical exam findings of a DRUJ injury?	DRUJ tenderness and DRUJ instability (piano key test)

Chapter 31
Distal Radius and Ulnar Fractures

Travis Blood

What test should be ordered on an elective basis after an elderly female has a distal radius fracture?	Dexa scan
After fixation of a distal radius fracture what joint needs to be checked for stability?	Distal radial-ulnar joint
What is the eponym of an extra-articular dorsally displaced distal radius?	Colles fracture
What is the eponym of an extra-articular volarly displaced distal radius?	Smiths fracture
What is the normal volar tilt of the distal radius?	11°
What is the acceptable volar tilt after reduction?	5° dorsal to 20° volar

(continued)

T. Blood, MD
Department of Orthopedics, Warren Alpert Medical School of
Brown University, Providence, RI, USA
e-mail: travis_blood@brown.edu

© Springer International Publishing AG, part of Springer Nature 2018   65
A. E. M. Eltorai et al. (eds.), *Essential Orthopedic Review*,
https://doi.org/10.1007/978-3-319-78387-1_31

(continued)

What is the acceptable articular step off?	2 mm
Do you have to fix associated ulnar styloid fractures?	Generally, these do not need to be fixed
What soft tissue structure attaches at the base of the ulnar styloid that can be injured during a distal radius fracture?	Triangular fibrocartilage complex
What nerve is compressed in acute carpal tunnel syndrome?	Median nerve

Chapter 32
Carpal Tunnel Syndrome

Andrew Paul Harris

Carpal tunnel syndrome is caused by neuropathy of what nerve?	Median nerve
What digits are most commonly affected by carpal tunnel syndrome?	Thumb, index, middle, and radial half of the ring finger
What are some conditions associated with a higher risk of developing carpal tunnel syndrome?	Diabetes, hypothyroidism, pregnancy, and obesity
Volar dislocation of what carpal bone is associated with acute carpal tunnel syndrome?	Lunate
What symptoms do patients with carpal tunnel syndrome often report?	Night pain, pins and needles, numbness, weakness, dropping objects (clumsiness)

(continued)

A. P. Harris, MD
Department of Orthopedic Surgery, Warren Alpert Medical School of Brown University, Providence, RI, USA

© Springer International Publishing AG, part of Springer Nature 2018
A. E. M. Eltorai et al. (eds.), *Essential Orthopedic Review*,
https://doi.org/10.1007/978-3-319-78387-1_32

(continued)

What nonsurgical treatments can be implemented to decrease symptoms?	Wrist night splints, corticosteroid injections
What ligament forms the roof of the carpal tunnel?	Transverse carpal ligament
What physical exam tests can be done to aid in the diagnosis of carpal tunnel syndrome?	Durkan's, phalen's, reverse phalen's, and tinel's tests
Night splints used to treat carpal tunnel syndrome should place the wrist in what position?	Neutral
What diagnostic test can be performed to determine the severity of median nerve neuropathy in carpal tunnel syndrome?	Electromyography and nerve conduction study (EMG/NCS)

Chapter 33
Cubital Tunnel Syndrome

Kalpit N. Shah

What is cubital tunnel syndrome (CuTS)?	Compression of the ulnar nerve around the elbow
What is the most common site of compression of the ulnar nerve?	Between the two heads of the flexor carpi ulnaris and its aponeurosis
What are sites of compression proximal to the medial epicondyle?	Arcade of Struthers (hiatus in the medial intermuscular septum) Medial intermuscular septum Osborne's fascia
What are sites of compression distal to the medial epicondyle?	Anconeus epitrochlearis Osborne's ligament (medial epicondyle to olecranon) Fascial bands of FCU Aponeurosis of FDS
What are common symptoms of CuTS?	Paresthesias of the small finger, ulnar half of the ring finger and ulnar dorsal hand, weak hand intrinsic muscles

(continued)

K. N. Shah, MD
Department of Orthopaedic Surgery, Warren Alpert School of Medicine, Brown University, Providence, RI, USA

© Springer International Publishing AG, part of Springer Nature 2018   69
A. E. M. Eltorai et al. (eds.), *Essential Orthopedic Review*,
https://doi.org/10.1007/978-3-319-78387-1_33

(continued)

What common hand functions are weaker in patients with CuTS?	Weakened grasp (intrinsic MCP flexors), weakened pinch (weak adductor pollicis)
What is the Froment's sign?	Due to weak adductor pollicis, the FPL fires to flex the thumb IP joint during key pinch (tested with a piece of paper in clinic)
Provocative tests for CuTS?	Tinel (tapping) sign at the elbow, elbow flexion >60s, direct pressure over elbow
What advanced testing may be obtained to confirm the diagnosis?	Electromyography or nerve conduction study
Nonoperative options?	Night splint with elbow at 45° flexion, forearm in neutral rotation
Surgical options for management of CuTS?	In situ decompression, subcutaneous or submuscular transposition of the ulnar nerve
What superficial nerve is at risk of injury during ulnar nerve surgery?	Medial antebrachial cutaneous nerve

Chapter 34
Other Compressive Neuropathies

Ross Feller

What are the classically described sites of suprascapular nerve entrapment and compression?	Entrapment occurs beneath the superior transverse scapular ligament within the suprascapular notch, whereas compression classically results from a posterior spinoglenoid notch cyst
How can one differentiate between these two sites of compression with physical examination?	Atrophy and weakness will involve both the supraspinatus (abduction) and infraspinatus (external rotation) with entrapment of the nerve in the suprascapular notch, whereas only the infraspinatus will be affected with more distal compression of the suprascapular nerve (i.e., isolated external rotation weakness will result)
What nerve is affected in pronator syndrome?	Median nerve

(continued)

R. Feller, MD
The Warren Alpert Medical School of Brown University,
Providence, RI, USA
e-mail: rjfell.ross@gmail.com

© Springer International Publishing AG, part of Springer Nature 2018   71
A. E. M. Eltorai et al. (eds.), *Essential Orthopedic Review*,
https://doi.org/10.1007/978-3-319-78387-1_34

(continued)

What are the various sites of compression (5) in pronator syndrome?	Supracondylar process of the humerus, ligament of Struthers, bicipital aponeurosis (lacertus fibrosus), between ulnar and humeral heads of pronator teres, FDS aponeurotic arch
What physical exam maneuvers can be employed to diagnosis pronator syndrome?	Tinel's at the anterior forearm (not the wrist as with CTS)
	Reproduction of symptoms with: (1) resisted elbow flexion and supination (compression at lacertus fibrosus), (2) resisted forearm pronation with elbow extended (compression between pronator heads), and (3) resisted MF flexion (compression at FDS fibrous arch)
What nerve is involved in radial tunnel syndrome?	Posterior interosseous nerve (PIN)
What are the potential sites of compression in radial tunnel syndrome?	Fibrous bands anterior to radiocapitellar joint, leach of Henry (radial recurrent vessels), medial edge of ECRB, arcade of Frohse (proximal aponeurotic/tendinous arch of supinator, most common), distal edge of supinator
What nerve is affected in Guyon's canal compression? Where does the nerve lie in relation to the artery?	Ulnar nerve at the level of the wrist/hand. Nerve is ulnar to artery
What are the boundaries of Guyon's canal?	Transverse carpal ligament/hypothenar muscles (floor), volar carpal ligament (roof), pisiform/pisohamate ligament (ulnar), hook of hamate (radial)
What are the zones of Guyon's canal?	Zone I is proximal to bifurcation of ulnar nerve (mixed motor and sensory), zone II surrounds deep motor branch, and zone III surrounds superficial sensory branch

Chapter 35
Kienbock's Disease

Devan Patel

What is the primary pathophysiology that is thought to cause Kienbock's disease?	Avascular necrosis of the lunate leading to eventual collapse; seen radiographically
What are the stages of Kienbock's disease seen radiographically?	Stage I—Typically no radiographic findings, possibly fractures seen, and changes on MRI Stage II—Sclerosis of the lunate with possible fragmentation Stage III—Fragmentation with collapse Stage IV—Degeneration of joint surfaces surrounding the lunate causing arthritis

(continued)

D. Patel, MD
Department of Orthopaedic Surgery, Warren Alpert Medical School of Brown University, Providence, RI, USA
e-mail: Devan_Patel@brown.edu

© Springer International Publishing AG, part of Springer Nature 2018   73
A. E. M. Eltorai et al. (eds.), *Essential Orthopedic Review*,
https://doi.org/10.1007/978-3-319-78387-1_35

(continued)

What is the typical history of a patient with Kienbock's disease?	Dorsal wrist pain over the lunate with a history of minor or repetitive trauma
What is the natural history of Kienbock's disease?	Progressive pain, decrease range of motion at the wrist, decreased grip strength, progressive arthritis
What are surgical options to treat this disease?	Joint pinning, joint leveling, radial osteotomy, proximal row carpectomy (PRC), joint fusions, revascularization procedures, and total wrist arthroplasty
What is the classic radiographic risk factor for those with Kienbock's disease?	Ulnar negative variance

Chapter 36
De Quervain's Tenosynovitis

Jeremy E. Raducha

Where is the location of pain in de Quervain's tenosynovitis?	Dorsoradial wrist
Which wrist compartment is involved?	First dorsal compartment of the wrist
Which tendons run in this compartment?	Extensor pollicis brevis and abductor pollicis longus

(continued)

Wolfe SWM. Tendinopathy. In: Wolfe SWM, editor. Green's operative hand surgery. 7th ed. Philadelphia: Elsevier; 2017. p. 1904–24. https://www-clinicalkey-com.revproxy.brown.edu/service/content/pdf/watermarked/3-s2.0-B9781455774272000563.pdf?locale=en_US. Accessed 18 Apr 2017.

Ilyas AM, Ast M, Schaffer AA, Thoder JM. de Quervain Tenosynovitis of the wrist. J Am Acad Orthop Surg. 2007;15(12):757–64. http://journals.lww.com/jaaos/Abstract/2007/12000/de_Quervain_Tenosynovitis_of_the_Wrist.9.aspx. Accessed 28 May 2017.

J. E. Raducha, MD
Department of Orthopaedic Surgery, Warren Alpert Medical School of Brown University, Providence, RI, USA

© Springer International Publishing AG, part of Springer Nature 2018   75
A. E. M. Eltorai et al. (eds.), *Essential Orthopedic Review*,
https://doi.org/10.1007/978-3-319-78387-1_36

(continued)

What is the classical physical exam maneuver that suggests de Quervain's if positive?	Finkelstein test or Eichhoff maneuver
What are the nonoperative options for treatment?	Rest, NSAIDs, bracing, corticosteroid injection
What is the surgical option for treatment?	Release of the first dorsal compartment
Which nerve is most at risk during surgical intervention?	Superficial branch of the radial nerve
What is the common reason for failed operative intervention?	Failure to decompress the extensor pollicis brevis subsheath

Chapter 37
Dupuytren's Disease

Andrew Paul Harris

What cells play a primary role in Dupuytren's disease?	Myofibroblasts
What two fingers are most commonly involved with Dupuytren's disease?	Small and ring fingers
What physical exam test can be used to determine severity of Dupuytren's disease?	Palm to table test
What type of enzyme may be injected to treat Dupuytren's disease?	Collagenase
Contracture of what tissue is the cause of Dupuytren's disease?	Fascia

(continued)

A. P. Harris, MD
Department of Orthopedic Surgery, Warren Alpert Medical School of Brown University, Providence, RI, USA
e-mail: andrew_harris@brown.edu

© Springer International Publishing AG, part of Springer Nature 2018   77
A. E. M. Eltorai et al. (eds.), *Essential Orthopedic Review*,
https://doi.org/10.1007/978-3-319-78387-1_37

(continued)

Fascial bands become cords in Dupuytren's disease. What cords may develop?	Pretendinous cord, spiral cord, natatory cord, retrovascular cord
The spiral cord causes the neurovascular bundle to displace in what direction?	Centrally and superficial to the A-1 pulley
What is the most common surgical treatment for Dupuytren's disease?	Fasciectomy
What is the most common complication of Dupuytren's surgical excision?	Wound edge necrosis, hematoma formation
In Dupuytren's disease, the thickening of tissue on the dorsum of the PIP joints is known as what?	Garrod's pads (knuckle pads)

Chapter 38
Trigger Finger

Andrew Paul Harris

Adult trigger finger is most often associated with what flexor tendon pulley?	A–1
Treatment of trigger finger with corticosteroid injection is less effective in what patient population?	Diabetics
What symptoms do patients with trigger finger often report?	Pain over the A–1 pulley, catching, locking of the affected digit
Pediatric trigger finger may be treated with surgical release of what structures?	A–1 pulley and also one slip of the flexor digitorum superficialis tendon

(continued)

A. P. Harris, MD
Department of Orthopedic Surgery, Warren Alpert Medical School of Brown University, Providence, RI, USA
e-mail: andrew_harris@brown.edu

© Springer International Publishing AG, part of Springer Nature 2018   79
A. E. M. Eltorai et al. (eds.), *Essential Orthopedic Review*,
https://doi.org/10.1007/978-3-319-78387-1_38

(continued)

Proximal to the A–1 pulley, what other structure may contribute to trigger finger?	Palmar aponeurosis pulley (also known as Manske's pulley)
What is the medical term to describe trigger finger?	Stenosing tenosynovitis
What are some medical conditions that may contribute to trigger finger?	Gout, rheumatoid arthritis, diabetes, trauma
What are two nonsurgical method of treating trigger finger?	Splinting, corticosteroid injection
What nerve is at risk for injury during surgical release of the thumb A–1 pulley?	Radial digital nerve to the thumb
A thickened nodule on the flexor tendon is known as what?	Notta's node or nodule

Chapter 39
Scaphoid Fractures

Andrew Paul Harris

What is the most common type of scaphoid fracture?	Waist fracture (middle third)
What direction is the blood flow to the scaphoid?	Retrograde
What scaphoid fracture is most prone to nonunion or avascular necrosis?	Proximal pole scaphoid fracture
Nonunion of the scaphoid may result in what chronic arthritic condition of the wrist?	Scaphoid nonunion advanced collapse (SNAC wrist)
Scaphoid fracture may be associated with dislocation of what carpal bone?	Lunate

(continued)

A. P. Harris, MD
Department of Orthopedic Surgery, Warren Alpert Medical School of Brown University, Providence, RI, USA
e-mail: andrew_harris@brown.edu

© Springer International Publishing AG, part of Springer Nature 2018   81
A. E. M. Eltorai et al. (eds.), *Essential Orthopedic Review*,
https://doi.org/10.1007/978-3-319-78387-1_39

(continued)

If a scaphoid fracture is suspected but not seen on radiographs, what additional imaging tests can be used?	CT scan or MRI (more sensitive)
What physical exam findings are associated with scaphoid fracture?	Tenderness with palpation of the snuff box and scaphoid tubercle
What implants may be used to surgically treat scaphoid fractures?	Headless compression screws, scaphoid plate
What is the most common cause of scaphoid fracture?	Fall with hyperextension of the wrist
If a nonunion of a scaphoid is suspected after fixation, what imaging test can be used to confirm?	CT-scan

Chapter 40
Other Carpal Bone Fractures

Devan Patel

Which patients classically get hook of the hamate fractures?	Those with trauma directly to the hand such as baseball players, hockey players, and golfers
Which tendons are closest to the hook and can cause pain when used?	The fourth and fifth FDP tendons
What radiographic view is important to obtain with hook of the hamate fractures?	Carpal tunnel view
What is the most common fracture mechanism of the triquetrum?	Ulnar styloid impaction on the triquetrum during forceful wrist extension

(continued)

D. Patel, MD
Department of Orthopaedic Surgery, Warren Alpert Medical School of Brown University, Providence, RI, USA
e-mail: Devan_Patel@brown.edu

© Springer International Publishing AG, part of Springer Nature 2018   83
A. E. M. Eltorai et al. (eds.), *Essential Orthopedic Review*,
https://doi.org/10.1007/978-3-319-78387-1_40

(continued)

What is the most common treatment for triquetrum fractures?	Splint or cast immobilization
Hypothenar tenderness can indicate a fracture of what carpal bone?	Pisiform
What are the two types of trapezium fractures?	Trapezial ridge fractures and trapezial body fractures
What type of trapezium fracture is commonly seen in cyclist?	Trapezial body fractures due to axial loading during a fall

Chapter 41
Lunate and Perilunate Dislocations

Andrew Paul Harris

What emergency condition may present with perilunate and lunate dislocations requiring emergency reduction and surgery?	Acute carpal tunnel syndrome
How many stages are in the Mayfield classification of perilunate/lunate dislocation?	Four stages
What three arcs may be injured to cause perilunate or lunate dislocations?	Greater arc, lesser arc, tranlunate arc
What is the most common carpal bone fracture associated with a perilunate dislocation?	Scaphoid (known as a transcaphoid perilunate dislocation)

(continued)

A. P. Harris, MD
Department of Orthopedic Surgery,
Warren Alpert Medical School of Brown University,
Providence, RI, USA
e-mail: andrew_harris@brown.edu

© Springer International Publishing AG, part of Springer Nature 2018   85
A. E. M. Eltorai et al. (eds.), *Essential Orthopedic Review*,
https://doi.org/10.1007/978-3-319-78387-1_41

(continued)

What carpal bone fractures may be associated with perilunate or lunate dislocations?	Radial styloid, scaphoid, capitate, triquetrum
What is the first stage of lesser arc perilunate/lunate dislocation?	Scapholunate ligament disruption
What is the second stage of lesser arc perilunate/lunate dislocation?	Disruption of the capitolunate articulation
What is the third stage of lesser arc perilunate/lunate dislocation	Disruption of the lunotriquetral ligament
What is the fourth stage of injury required to produce a complete lunate dislocation?	Disruption of the short radiolunate ligaments causing failure of the radiolunate articulation
What radiograph is best used to diagnosis a perilunate or lunate dislocation?	Lateral wrist radiograph

Chapter 42
First Metacarpal Base Fracture

Travis Blood

What are the deforming forces of the Bennett fracture?	Abductor pollicis longus, extensor pollicis longus and adductor pollicis—adduction and supination
What is the volar lip of the first metacarpal attached to in a Bennett fracture?	Volar oblique ligament
What X-ray view is used to best visualize the first metacarpal base fracture?	Hyperpronated thumb view
Does the Bennett or the Rolando fracture have a better prognosis?	Bennett fracture

T. Blood, MD
Brown University Orthopedics, Brown University,
Providence, RI, USA
e-mail: travis_blood@brown.edu

© Springer International Publishing AG, part of Springer Nature 2018   87
A. E. M. Eltorai et al. (eds.), *Essential Orthopedic Review*,
https://doi.org/10.1007/978-3-319-78387-1_42

Chapter 43
Skier's or Gamekeeper's Thumb

Steven F. DeFroda

What is a skier's thumb?	Acute injury to the thumb metacarpophalangeal (MCP) joint ulnar collateral ligament (UCL)
How does gamekeeper's thumb differ?	This is a chronic attenuation of the UCL (as opposed to an acute rupture)
What tendon can get interposed in the ligament tear?	Adductor pollicus aponeurosis
What is the eponym for an interposed adductor tendon in a UCL injury?	"Stener" lesion

(continued)

S. F. DeFroda, MD, ME
Department of Orthopaedic Surgery, Warren Alpert Medical School of Brown University, Providence, RI, USA

© Springer International Publishing AG, part of Springer Nature 2018   89
A. E. M. Eltorai et al. (eds.), *Essential Orthopedic Review*,
https://doi.org/10.1007/978-3-319-78387-1_43

(continued)

What are the operative indications?	>20° variation on varus/valgus stress >35° of opening at neutral, or 30° of MCP flexion
What is the mechanism of injury?	Hyperextension and abduction at the MCP joint
What type of imaging can aid in diagnosis?	Stress radiographs of the MCP joint looking for widening

References

1. Schroeder NS, Goldfarb CA. Thumb ulnar collateral and radial collateral ligament injuries. Clin Sports Med. 2015;34(1):117–26. https://doi.org/10.1016/j.csm.2014.09.004.

Chapter 44
Boxer's Fracture

Devan Patel

What are the most common metacarpals to have a boxer's fracture?	Fourth and fifth metacarpals
What is the most common deformity? What muscles cause this deformity?	Interossei muscles cause apex dorsal deformity
What radiographs are commonly used to measure the deformity of these fractures?	True lateral radiographs are able to depict the sagittal plane deformity
Why are the fourth and fifth digits able to tolerate increased angulation well?	Increased range of motion at the metacarpal phalangeal joint

(continued)

D. Patel, MD
Department of Orthopaedic Surgery, Warren Alpert Medical
School of Brown University, Providence, RI, USA
e-mail: Devan_Patel@brown.edu

© Springer International Publishing AG, part of Springer Nature 2018 91
A. E. M. Eltorai et al. (eds.), *Essential Orthopedic Review*,
https://doi.org/10.1007/978-3-319-78387-1_44

(continued)

What is the most common complication of conservative treatment?	Stiffness and prominence in the palm
What are the operative indications for this type of fracture?	Open fractures, unstable fractures, volar angulation greater than 10–50° depending on the digit, significant rotational deformity
What are some surgical options for fixations?	Dorsal plating, intramedullary fixation, lag screw fixation, and percutaneous pinning

Chapter 45
Phalangeal Fractures

Kalpit N. Shah

Which phalanx is the most commonly fractured?	Distal phalanx
What deformity is created in proximal phalanx fractures? Why?	Apex volar – Proximal fragment is flexed due to interossei – Distal fragment is extended due to central slip
What deformity is created in middle phalanx fractures? Why?	– Apex dorsal (if fracture is proximal to FDS insertion)—central slip extends the proximal fragment and FDS flexes the distal fragment – Apex volar (if fracture is distal to FDS insertion)—FDS flexes the proximal fragment

(continued)

K. N. Shah, MD
Department of Orthopaedic Surgery, Warren Alpert School
of Medicine of Brown University, Providence, RI, USA

© Springer International Publishing AG, part of Springer Nature 2018   93
A. E. M. Eltorai et al. (eds.), *Essential Orthopedic Review*,
https://doi.org/10.1007/978-3-319-78387-1_45

(continued)

What are the operative indications for a proximal or middle phalanx fracture?	Extra-articular, <10° angulation, and 2 mm shortening
What are the operative indications for a distal phalanx fracture?	Nail bed injury associated with a distal phalanx fracture
What is the most common complication of phalangeal fractures?	Stiffness of the affected digit

Chapter 46
Finger (Phalangeal) Dislocations

Tyler S. Pidgeon

Which proximal interphalangeal (PIP) joint dislocation type is most common?	Dorsal
What soft tissue structures are injured during a dorsal PIP joint dislocation?	The volar plate and at least one collateral ligament
What deformity results from untreated dorsal PIP joint dislocations?	Swan neck deformity
What soft tissue structures are injured during a volar PIP joint dislocation?	The central slip and at least one collateral ligament

(continued)

T. S. Pidgeon, MD
Department of Orthopaedic Surgery, The Warren Alpert Medical School at Brown University, Providence, RI, USA

© Springer International Publishing AG, part of Springer Nature 2018   95
A. E. M. Eltorai et al. (eds.), *Essential Orthopedic Review*,
https://doi.org/10.1007/978-3-319-78387-1_46

(continued)

What deformity results from untreated volar PIP joint dislocations?	Boutonniere deformity
How are dorsal PIP dislocations treated?	Closed reduction and buddy-taping for 3–6 weeks. To reduce apply volar-directed force on the middle phalanx. Hyperextension of the middle phalanx prior to volar force may be required. Pulling traction on the finger causes the volar plate to block reduction. Open reduction with volar plate extraction may be required in irreducible dislocations
How are volar PIP dislocations treated?	Closed reduction and extension splinting for 6–8 weeks
Describe the anatomy of a rotary PIP dislocation.	One proximal phalanx condyle buttholes between the central slip and lateral band
How are rotatory PIP dislocations reduced?	Closed reduction is attempted with finger traction with metacarpophalangeal and PIP joints at 90° of flexion to relax the lateral band. However, open reduction is required in most cases
How are dorsal distal interphalangeal (DIP) joint dislocations treated?	Closed reduction and immobilization in slight flexion for 2 weeks via a dorsal splint. Open reduction may be required if volar plate is interposed

Chapter 47
Metacarpal Fractures

Tyler S. Pidgeon

What are the acceptable parameters for nonoperative management of finger metacarpal shaft fractures?	No rotational deformity. No more than 2–5 mm of shortening. Maximum of 10–20° of angulation at the index and long fingers, 30° of angulation at the ring finger, and 40° of angulation at the small finger
Why does shaft angulation acceptability differ between fingers?	There is greater carpometacarpal (CMC) joint range of motion at the small and ring fingers compared to the middle and index fingers
What are indications for surgical management of finger metacarpal fractures?	Open fractures, intra-articular fractures, rotational malalignment, displacement as listed above, multiple metacarpal fractures, border digit fractures

(continued)

T. S. Pidgeon, MD
Department of Orthopaedic Surgery, The Warren Alpert Medical School at Brown University, Providence, RI, USA

© Springer International Publishing AG, part of Springer Nature 2018   97
A. E. M. Eltorai et al. (eds.), *Essential Orthopedic Review*,
https://doi.org/10.1007/978-3-319-78387-1_47

(continued)

How should hands with metacarpal fractures be immobilized?	In intrinsic plus position to tighten the collateral ligaments of the metacarpophalangeal (MCP) joint via the cam effect of the metacarpal head; thus, preventing MCP stiffness
What are surgical options of metacarpal shaft fractures?	Closed reduction and percutaneous pinning, open reduction and internal fixation (ORIF) with a plate, ORIF with lag screws (minimum of two), tension band wiring, cerclage/interosseous wiring, external fixation, open intramedullary fixation
What are the acceptable parameters for nonoperative management of finger metacarpal neck fractures?	No rotational deformity. No more than 2–5 mm of shortening. Maximum of 10–15° of angulation at the index and long fingers, 30–40° of angulation at the ring finger, and 50–60° of angulation at the small finger
Name and describe the reduction technique for metacarpal neck fractures.	The Jahss Technique: Flex the MCP joint to 90° and apply dorsally directed force to the metacarpal head via the proximal phalanx while stabilizing the metacarpal shaft

Chapter 48
Traumatic/Revision Finger Amputation

P. Kaveh Mansuripur

When feasible, what coverage technique provides the best 2-point discrimination?	Healing by secondary intention (granulation)
What kind of pain do patients most often complain about?	Cold intolerance
The "composite graft" technique works best in which patients?	Children
In general, what kind of suture should be used in the fingertips?	Absorbable monofilament (gut, chromic, etc.)
A "V-Y" flap is useful in what kind of tissue loss?	Transverse or dorsal oblique

(continued)

P. Kaveh Mansuripur, MD
Hand and Upper Limb Surgery, Stanford University School of Medicine, Stanford, CA, USA

© Springer International Publishing AG, part of Springer Nature 2018
A. E. M. Eltorai et al. (eds.), *Essential Orthopedic Review*,
https://doi.org/10.1007/978-3-319-78387-1_48

(continued)

What is the most common complication of the thenar flap in adults?	PIP flexion contracture
The Moberg flap is used for which digit?	The thumb
What is the mechanism of a lumbrical plus finger?	In amputations proximal to the FDP insertion, attempt at finger flexion will tension the lumbricals and cause paradoxical extension
What are the major goals in treating traumatic digit amputations?	Cover bone, maintain length, maximize sensation, prevent neuromas, maximize range of motion and function
When revising a traumatic amputation, how are neuromas prevented?	Cut digital nerves under tension so that they retract

Chapter 49
Tears of the TFCC

Avi DeLano Goodman

What are the components of the TFCC?	Dorsal and volar radioulnar ligaments, central articular disc, meniscus homolog, ulnar collateral ligament, ECU subsheath, ulnolunate and ulnotriquetral ligaments
Which areas are vascularized?	Periphery (10–40%), while central is avascular (similar to the meniscus)
What are the symptoms and physical exam findings?	Ulnar-sided wrist pain, especially with turning a key (rotation), and ulnar or radial deviation
What are the X-ray views needed to evaluate?	3-view hand, 3-view wrist — usually negative, but zero-rotation PA will show ulnar variance

(continued)

A. D. Goodman, MD
Department of Orthopaedics, Warren Alpert Medical School
of Brown University, Providence, RI, USA
e-mail: avi_goodman@brown.edu

© Springer International Publishing AG, part of Springer Nature 2018   101
A. E. M. Eltorai et al. (eds.), *Essential Orthopedic Review*,
https://doi.org/10.1007/978-3-319-78387-1_49

(continued)

Which is the best imaging study for TFCC evaluation?	MR arthrogram, with sensitivity 84% and specificity 85%
What is the gold standard for diagnosis?	Wrist arthroscopy
What are the classifications?	Class 1—traumatic Class 2—degenerative (Subtypes describe location)
What are the surgical options?	Arthroscopic debridement, repair, ulnar shaft shortening, limited ulnar head resection

Chapter 50
Carpal Instability

Avi DeLano Goodman

What are the broad classifications of instability?	Dissociative (within a carpal row or intracarpal) Nondissociative (between carpal and intercarpal rows) and combined (both)
What are the types of dissociative instability?	DISI (from scapholunate tears → scaphoid flexes and lunate becomes dorsally angulated) and VISI (volar intercalated segmental instability, from lunotriquetral tears → lunate flexes with scaphoid and becomes volarly angulated)
What is the classification of perilunate injuries?	Mayfield (I–IV)
What are the X-ray findings?	Disruption of Gilula's arcs

(continued)

A. D. Goodman, MD
Department of Orthopaedics, Warren Alpert Medical School
of Brown University, Providence, RI, USA
e-mail: avi_goodman@brown.edu

© Springer International Publishing AG, part of Springer Nature 2018   103
A. E. M. Eltorai et al. (eds.), *Essential Orthopedic Review*,
https://doi.org/10.1007/978-3-319-78387-1_50

(continued)

Clinically, what is the acute concern with perilunate dissociation?	Acute carpal tunnel syndrome
What is the surgical option for perilunate dissociation?	Urgent reduction and fixation, with possible carpal tunnel release
What are the surgical options for chronic instability?	Radial styloidectomy, denervation, proximal row carpectomy, partial or complete wrist fusion

Chapter 51
Flexor Tendon Injuries

Andrew D. Sobel

Describe the flexor tendon "zones"	In the fingers
	Zone 1—distal to FDS insertion
	Zone 2 ("no man's land")—distal to distal palmar crease (A1 pulley), proximal to FDS insertion
	Zone 3—distal to carpal tunnel, proximal to distal palmar crease (A1 pulley)
	Zone 4—Within carpal tunnel
	Zone 5—Wrist and forearm proximal to carpal tunnel
	In the thumb
	Zone 1—Distal to interphalangeal joint (IP)
	Zone 2—Distal to A1 pulley, proximal to IP
	Zone 3—Thenar eminence
	Zone 4–5—Same as fingers

(continued)

A. D. Sobel, MD
Department of Orthopedics, Warren Alpert Medical School of Brown University, Providence, RI, USA

© Springer International Publishing AG, part of Springer Nature 2018   105
A. E. M. Eltorai et al. (eds.), *Essential Orthopedic Review*,
https://doi.org/10.1007/978-3-319-78387-1_51

(continued)

Describe the flexor pulley system	Five annular pulleys, three cruciate pulleys prevent tendon bowstringing and direct tendon gliding
	Odd numbered pulleys (A1, A3, A5) overlay joints (metacarpophalangeal, proximal IP, distal IP) and arise from volar plate of joints
	Thumb has A1, Av, oblique, A2 pulleys only
Which pulleys are the most important to prevent flexor tendon bowstringing in the fingers? In the thumb?	Fingers—A2 and A4 Thumb—Oblique pulley
What is the orientation of flexor digitorum profundus (FDP) and flexor digitorum superficialis (FDS) tendons in the palm and digit and what is the anatomic landmark where the orientation changes?	Palm—FDP deep, FDS superficial Finger—FDP superficial, FDS deep FDS tendon splits at "campers chiasm" and dives deep to insert on middle phalanx around FDP which continues distal to insert on distal phalanx
What are the specific functions of the FDP and FDS tendons?	FDP—Flexion of distal IP joint FDS—Flexion of proximal IP joint

(continued)

What is the predominate way that tendons receive nutrition?	Diffusion through synovial fluid created by the tendon's synovial sheath
When can flexor tendon lacerations be treated nonoperatively?	Laceration of <60% tendon width
What is the most important determinant of flexor tendon laceration suture repair strength?	Number of suture strands crossing repair site
Besides crossing sutures, what can be done to improve gliding and strength of a repaired tendon?	Simple, running epitendinous suture
How are chronic flexor tendon injuries typically treated?	Two-stage reconstruction Stage 1—Silicone rod placement Stage 2—Tendon graft interposition

Chapter 52
Extensor Tendon Injuries

Devan Patel

Which is the most frequently injured zone?	Zone VI
What is a zone I injury and what is the resulting deformity?	Injury at or distal to the DIP joint, causing a mallet finger deformity
What is a zone III injury and what is the resulting deformity?	Disruption of the tendon over the proximal interphalangeal joint causing a central slip injury and a boutonniere deformity
What zone is a "fight bite" injury and what is the treatment?	Zone V, over the metacarpal phalangeal joint. Treatment is typically irrigation and debridement

(continued)

D. Patel, MD
Department of Orthopaedic Surgery, Warren Alpert Medical School of Brown University, Providence, RI, USA
e-mail: Devan_Patel@brown.edu

© Springer International Publishing AG, part of Springer Nature 2018   109
A. E. M. Eltorai et al. (eds.), *Essential Orthopedic Review*,
https://doi.org/10.1007/978-3-319-78387-1_52

(continued)

What is the Elson's test and what does it indicate?	The patient's finger is position at 90° at the PIP, typically over the corner of a table. The patient is asked to extend against resistance. Normal: PIP extension with a flexible DIP. Abnormal: No PIP extension, with rigid DIP. Indicates central slip injury
What is the classic nonoperative treatment of extensor injuries?	Extension splitting
What are operative options for extensor tendon injuries?	Tendon repair, tendon reconstruction, and tendon transfers
Nondisplaced distal radius fractures can result in what extensor tendon injury?	Extensor pollicis longus rupture
What is the typically treatment for an EPL rupture?	EIP to EPL tendon transfer

Chapter 53
Nerve Injury

Ross Feller

Describe the relationship between the digital artery and nerve at the level of the (1) palm and (2) middle phalanx?	In the palm, the artery lies superficial (volar) to the nerve, whereas at the level of the middle phalanx, this relationship is reversed
Name the different connective tissue layers of a nerve.	Epineurium, perineurium, endoneurium
Describe the different three main categories of nerve injury.	Neuropraxia—No structural/anatomic change to the nerve, best prognosis; Axonotmesis—Perineurium remains intact but axons within a fascicle rupture, prognosis based on degree of scarring within the fiber; Neurotmesis—Complete nerve rupture, requires repair or reconstruction

(continued)

R. Feller, MD
The Warren Alpert Medical School of Brown University,
Providence, RI, USA
e-mail: rjfell.ross@gmail.com

© Springer International Publishing AG, part of Springer Nature 2018   111
A. E. M. Eltorai et al. (eds.), *Essential Orthopedic Review*,
https://doi.org/10.1007/978-3-319-78387-1_53

(continued)

What is the percentage of nerve stretch that leads to neuropraxia and axonotmesis?	The nerve can tolerated up to 10% of stretch, with 15% leading to neuropraxic injury and 20% or greater leading to axonotmesis
What is one reliable method for determining digital nerve continuity in the uncooperative child or the unconscious patient?	Water immersion testing: Presence of wrinkling or puckering of the finger within 4 min of submerging under water at 40 °C
What is the rate of growth of a peripheral nerve following repair?	One millimeter per day or 1 in. per month
What is one way to track recovery of an axonotmetic nerve injury using physical examination?	Presence of an advancing Tinel's sign along the path of the injured nerve
What is the most common nerve injury resulting from low-energy gunshot wounds? What is the significance of this in terms of treatment?	Neuropraxia, therefore most low energy gunshot wounds can be managed with observation and not acute exploration
What are the available techniques for direct end-to-end nerve repair? Which technique is mostly used presently and what is the main reason proponents advocate for this technique?	Epineural and grouped fascicular repair. Epineural repair is used most commonly, with advocates believing that the additional intraneural damage involved in manipulating individual fascicles can lead to more scarring and worse clinical results
What other techniques are available for nerve repair other than direct end-to-end suturing?	Adhesives (e.g., Tisseel, Evicel, and DuraSeal), conduits (e.g., Axogen, vein graft), nerve grafts (autograft, allograft, or vascularized nerve graft), end-to-side neurorraphy, nerve transfers

(continued)

What is the "rule of 18"?	The number of inches from the site of nerve injury to the supplied muscle plus the number of months from injury should be less than 18 inch. order for primary nerve repair to be considered. The basis of this principal lies in the fact that motor end plates will become refractory to reinnervation after about 18 months in the adult patient

Chapter 54
Replantation

Steven F. DeFroda

What is the most important factor when considering replantation?	Mechanism of injury
What is the accepted warm ischemia time for replantation?	<6 h proximal to carpus, <12 h for digits
What is the accepted cold ischemia time for replantation?	<12 h proximal to carpus, <24 h for digits
How should an amputated digit be transported?	Wrapped in saline moistened gauze, in a sealed plastic bag, on ice
What are the indications for replantation?	<ul><li>Thumb</li><li>Through palm</li><li>Multiple digits</li><li>Wrist or proximal</li><li>Any level in children</li><li>Individual digits distal to flexor digitorum superficialis insertion</li></ul>
What is the generally accepted order for the repair of structures during replantation?	Bone, extensor tendon, artery, vein, flexor tendon, nerve, skin (BEAVFTNS)

(continued)

S. F. DeFroda, MD, ME
Department of Orthopaedic Surgery, Warren Alpert Medical School of Brown University, Providence, RI, USA

© Springer International Publishing AG, part of Springer Nature 2018   115
A. E. M. Eltorai et al. (eds.), *Essential Orthopedic Review*,
https://doi.org/10.1007/978-3-319-78387-1_54

(continued)

| What is the generally accepted order for replantation of multiple digits? | Thumb, long, ring, small, index |
| In a multiple digit replantation, is it preferred to repair digit-by-digit or structure-by-structure? | Structure-by-structure |

References

1. Beris AE, Lykissas MG, Korompilias AV, Mitsionis GI, Vekris MD, Kostas-Agnantis IP. Digit and hand replantation. Arch Orthop Trauma Surg. 2010;130(9):1141–7. https://doi.org/10.1007/s00402-009-1021-7.

Chapter 55
Rheumatoid Arthritis and Other Inflammatory Arthritides

Ross Feller

What is the classic radiographic pattern of arthropathy associated with psoriatic arthritis?	Pencil-in-cup deformity
What is arthritis mutilans and what are the classic findings associated with this disease?	Fulminant stage of osteolysis most commonly observed in severe psoriatic arthritis; osteolysis of all interphalangeal joints with digital collapse/shortening resulting in "opera glass hand"
What is the characteristic radiographic appearance of systemic lupus erythematosus (SLE)-related arthropathy?	Joint subluxation resembling RA without radiographic articular or bony destruction

(continued)

R. Feller, MD
The Warren Alpert Medical School of Brown University, Providence, RI, USA
e-mail: rjfell.ross@gmail.com

© Springer International Publishing AG, part of Springer Nature 2018   117
A. E. M. Eltorai et al. (eds.), *Essential Orthopedic Review*,
https://doi.org/10.1007/978-3-319-78387-1_55

(continued)

Define swan neck and boutonniere deformity?	Swan neck = PIP hyperextension, DIP flexion; Boutonniere = PIP hyperflexion, DIP extension
What is the difference in deformity in RA vs. psoriatic arthritis?	RA—MCP flexion and PIP extension (swan neck deformity), psoriatic arthritis—MCP hyperextension, PIP flexion (boutonniere)
What are the general guidelines for withholding of the various immunomodulating medications preoperatively?	Methotrexate and hydroxychloroquine: do not withhold; Cyclophosphamide, azathioprine, sulfasalazine: several days; Leflunomide: 2 weeks; DMARDs: two treatment cycles
What is the common deformity affecting the MCP joints in RA?	Volar and ulnar subluxation
What are the options available for correction of (1) passively correctable and (2) fixed MCP deformity related to RA?	Passively correctable deformity addressed with tendon realignment and soft tissue reconstruction; fixed deformity addressed with arthroplasty
What is caput ulna?	Chronic DRUJ involvement leads to destruction and dorsal subluxation of the ulna resulting in dorsal prominence, mechanical irritation of extensor tendons, and possible rupture
What the treatment options for single (small finger) and double extensor tendon (ring and small finger) rupture in RA?	Single—End to end repair, suture to adjacent tendon, graft; Double—Suture ring finger stump to intact middle finger extensor tendon, EIP transfer to small finger

Chapter 56
Degenerative Arthritis of the Hand and Wrist

Ross Feller

What is the ideal position of fusion of the thumb MCP?	10–20° flexion, 20 pronation, 20° abduction
What is the ideal position of fusion of the PIPJs?	Index finger 20–25 flexion, middle finger 30 flexion, ring finger 40 flexion, small finger 40–45 flexion
What is the ideal position of fusion of the DIPJs?	Neutral to slight flexion
What are the initial radiographic changes of SLAC wrist?	Beaking of the radial styloid with eventual radioscaphoid arthritis
What are the stages of SNAC?	I-radial styloid, radioscaphoid OA; II-scaphocapitate OA; III-periscaphoid OA

(continued)

R. Feller, MD
The Warren Alpert Medical School of Brown University,
Providence, RI, USA
e-mail: rjfell.ross@gmail.com

© Springer International Publishing AG, part of Springer Nature 2018   119
A. E. M. Eltorai et al. (eds.), *Essential Orthopedic Review*,
https://doi.org/10.1007/978-3-319-78387-1_56

(continued)

What is the key factor guiding the decision between performing proximal row carpectomy (PRC) versus four-corner arthrodesis (FCA) in the setting of SLAC wrist?	Status of the capitate and lunate facet articular cartilage
What staging system is commonly used in thumb CMC OA?	Eaton staging
What is the classic deformity associated with end-stage thumb CMC OA?	Metacarpal adduction with MCP hyperextension
What surgical treatment options are available for management of DRUJ OA?	Sauve-Kapandji, Darrach, ulnar hemiresection arthroplasty, implant arthroplasty

Chapter 57
Complex Regional Pain Syndrome

Ross Feller

What are the main symptoms of CRPS?	Swelling, pain, hyperesthesia/allodynia, sensory abnormalities, skin changes
What are the modalities available for diagnosis of CRPS other than history and physical examination?	Radiography (showing demineralization of the limb), triple phase bone scan, quantitative sweat test versus the contralateral limb, thermography, and diagnostic sympathetic nerve block
What changes occur in the transition to the chronic form of CRPS?	There is a transition from "warm CRPS," which is dominated by inflammatory symptoms, to "cold CRPS," characterized by autonomic dysfunction, atrophy, contractures, dystonia, hair/nail changes

(continued)

R. Feller, MD
The Warren Alpert Medical School of Brown University,
Providence, RI, USA
e-mail: rjfell.ross@gmail.com

© Springer International Publishing AG, part of Springer Nature 2018   121
A. E. M. Eltorai et al. (eds.), *Essential Orthopedic Review*,
https://doi.org/10.1007/978-3-319-78387-1_57

(continued)

What has been shown in some studies to decrease rates of CRPS following distal radius fracture?	Vitamin C
What are other available treatment options for CRPS?	Bisphosphonates, calcitonin, occupational therapy (graded motor imagery and mirror therapy), oral steroids, acupuncture, spinal cord stimulation, sympathectomy, and in some severe cases, amputation

Chapter 58
Hand Infections

Ross Feller

What is the definition of paronychia and felon?	A paronychia is an infection between the nail plate and eponychial fold. A felon is a suppurative infection of the pulp of the distal phalanx of a finger or thumb
What is the most common organism responsible for infection following a cat bite and a human bite?	Pasteurella multocida (cat bite) and Eikenella corrodens (human bite)
What is Parona's space?	The potential space of the volar distal forearm between the pronator quadratus and the sheath of the FDP tendons. It is in continuity with the midpalmar space
What are the three deep spaces of the hand?	Thenar, midpalmar, and hypothenar

(continued)

R. Feller, MD
The Warren Alpert Medical School of Brown University,
Providence, RI, USA
e-mail: rjfell.ross@gmail.com

© Springer International Publishing AG, part of Springer Nature 2018   123
A. E. M. Eltorai et al. (eds.), *Essential Orthopedic Review*,
https://doi.org/10.1007/978-3-319-78387-1_58

(continued)

What structures divide the thenar and midpalmar, and midpalmar and hypothenar spaces?	Midpalmar oblique septum (runs from palmar fascia to third metacarpal shaft) and hypothenar septum (palmar aponeurosis to fifth metacarpal shaft)
What is a collar button abscess? What is the classic position of the fingers with a collar button abscess?	An abscess of the interdigital web space. Fingers are held in an abducted position
What are Kanavel's signs?	Four signs associated with the clinical diagnosis of flexor tenosynovitis: (1) finger held in flexed posture, (2) fusiform swelling of the digit, (3) tenderness along the flexor sheath, (4) pain with passive extension of the finger
What are the signs and symptoms of necrotizing fasciitis?	Innocuous appearing or cellulitic with extreme tenderness (pain out of proportion) in early stages, with progression to bullae formation, soft tissue crepitus, hyper/anesthesia, and frank soft tissue necrosis accompanied by systemic sepsis as disease progresses
What are the most common organisms implicated in necrotizing fasciitis?	Type I-mixed anaerobic/aerobic including non-group A strep Type II-Group A strep
What is the organism responsible for gas gangrene?	Clostridium species

Part III
The Lower Extremity

Chapter 59
External Snapping Hip

John R. Tuttle

What anatomic structures are involved in external snapping hip?	Iliotibial band snapping over greater trochanter
Is external snapping hip usually painful?	No
Are radiographic and MRI findings typically normal in this condition?	Yes
What test helps diagnose a tight tensor fascia lata?	Ober's test
Is nonoperative treatment successful in most cases?	Yes
What is the surgical treatment for painful external snapping hip that fails nonoperative treatment?	IT band lengthening (or windowing)
What is a potential risk specific to this operation?	Trendelenburg gait

J. R. Tuttle, MD, MS
Sports Medicine, Department of Orthopaedic Surgery, Virginia
Tech Carilion School of Medicine, Roanoke, VA, USA
e-mail: jrtuttle@carilionclinic.org

© Springer International Publishing AG, part of Springer Nature 2018   127
A. E. M. Eltorai et al. (eds.), *Essential Orthopedic Review*,
https://doi.org/10.1007/978-3-319-78387-1_59

Bibliography

1. Lewis CL. Extra-articular snapping hip: a literature review. Sports Health. 2010;2(3):186–90. https://doi.org/10.1177/1941738109357298.

Chapter 60
Fractures of the Proximal Femur

Viorel Raducan

What is the most common mechanism of injury for fractures of the proximal femur in the elderly?	Fall from a standing height
What is the most common predisposing factor for fractures of the proximal femur?	Osteoporosis
What is the typical clinical finding in fractures of the proximal femur?	Shortening/external rotation and abduction
What are the most common orthopedic complications of fractures of the femoral neck?	Nonunion and osteonecrosis

(continued)

V. Raducan, MD, FRCS(C)
Department of Orthopaedic Surgery, Marshall University School of Medicine, Huntington, WV, USA
e-mail: raducan@marshall.edu

© Springer International Publishing AG, part of Springer Nature 2018   129
A. E. M. Eltorai et al. (eds.), *Essential Orthopedic Review*,
https://doi.org/10.1007/978-3-319-78387-1_60

(continued)

What is the preferred treatment for fractures of the proximal femur?	Surgery
What is the major benefit of surgical treatment in fractures of the proximal femur?	Decreased mortality at 1 year after fracture
What is the most useful imaging study for fractures of the proximal femur?	X-rays—hip (AP/lateral), pelvis (AP), full length femur (AP/lateral)
What is the prerequisite for optimal outcome of surgery for proximal femur fractures?	Optimization of the medical status and timing (within 48 h of injury)
What are the most common methods of surgical treatment for fractures of the femoral neck?	Internal fixation (if undisplaced) and arthroplasty (if displaced)
What is a stable intertrochanteric fracture?	Absence of fracture in the lesser trochanter (the calcar)
What is an unstable intertrochanteric fracture?	Presence of fracture of the calcar and/or reverse obliquity fracture line (proximal medial to distal and lateral)
What is the method of treatment for stable intertrochanteric fractures?	Dynamic hip screw or cephalomedullary nail (equal results)
What is the preferred method of treatment for unstable intertrochanteric fractures?	Cephalomedullary nail (prevents shortening and varus malunions)
What is the most common complication in surgical treatment of intertrochanteric fracture?	Screw cutout
What are the predictors of increased mortality after surgery for proximal femur fracture in the elderly?	Male sex, age over 85, delay of surgery (>48 h), > 2 comorbidities, ASA III–IV, intertrochanteric pattern

(continued)

What is the position of malunions in proximal femur fractures?	VARUS ± shortening ± external rotation
What are the characteristics of atypical femur fractures?	Low energy/transverse/no comminution/incomplete/ biphosphphonate use
What is the most sensitive/ specific imaging study for the diagnosis of undisplaced fractures of the proximal femur with negative X-rays?	MRI scan
What is a subtrochanteric fracture?	Fracture of the proximal femur below the lesser trochanter (with possible proximal/distal extension)
What is the treatment of subtrochanteric fractures?	Surgery—internal fixation. Exception—contraindication general/regional anesthesia

Chapter 61
Native Hip Dislocations

Viorel Raducan

What is the incidence of hip dislocations?	Hip dislocations are rare injuries
What are the most potent characteristics of hip dislocations?	High energy trauma in young patients with 95% incidence of associated injuries
How are hip dislocations classified?	Position of the head in relationship with the acetabulum (anterior/posterior) and presence of associated injuries (complex—with associated injuries, simple—no associated injuries)
What is the incidence of posterior hip dislocations?	90.0%

(continued)

V. Raducan, MD, FRCS(C)
Department of Orthopaedic Surgery, Marshall University School of Medicine, Huntington, WV, USA
e-mail: raducan@marshall.edu

© Springer International Publishing AG, part of Springer Nature 2018   133
A. E. M. Eltorai et al. (eds.), *Essential Orthopedic Review*,
https://doi.org/10.1007/978-3-319-78387-1_61

(continued)

What is the mechanism of posterior hip dislocation?	Dashboard injury (impact on the knee with the hip adducted and internally rotated)
What are the associated injuries in posterior hip dislocations?	Fractures of the posterior wall of the acetabulum, femoral head and neck, injury to the sciatic nerve, fractures around the knee (25%)
What is the clinical presentation in posterior?	Leg shortened, hip flexed, adducted, and internally rotated
What is the determinant prognostic factor in treatment of hip dislocation?	EMERGENT REDUCTION—within 6 h of injury/presentation
What are the imaging studies?	X-rays—AP pelvis and CT scan
What are the indications for CT scan in hip dislocations?	Postreduction, complex dislocations
What is the mechanism of anterior hip dislocations?	Impact on the leg in abduction
What is the classification of anterior hip dislocation?	SUPERIOR (impact on the leg in abduction and extension) and INFERIOR (obturator)—impact on the leg in hip flexion, abduction, and external rotation
What are the indications of open reduction in hip dislocation?	Irreducible dislocation, nonconcentric reduction, intra-articular body, complex dislocations

(continued)

What are the associated injuries in anterior hip dislocations?	Femoral head impaction and chondral injuries
What are the complications of hip dislocations?	Osteonecrosis of the femoral head (5–40%), posttraumatic arthritis (20%), sciatic nerve palsy (8–20%), recurrent dislocation (<2%)
How can hip dislocations be differentiated clinically?	The position of the hip (internal rotation–POSTERIOR, external rotation–ANTERIOR)

Chapter 62
Hip Osteoarthritis

Stephen Marcaccio

Define osteoarthritis.	A pathologic, non-reversible condition characterized by destruction of articular cartilage
Describe a physical exam for a patient with hip OA.	Overweight body habitus, potential leg length discrepancy, lack of full extension or flexion in passive ROM, catching/clicking
Name four radiographic findings with OA.	1. Subchondral cysts 2. Subchondral sclerosis 3. Osteophyte formation 4. Joint space narrowing
What is the conservative treatment for hip OA?	Physical therapy, scheduled anti-inflammatories, weight loss

(continued)

S. Marcaccio, MD
Department of Orthopaedic Surgery, Rhode Island Hospital, Brown University, Providence, RI, USA
e-mail: stephen_marcaccio@brown.edu

© Springer International Publishing AG, part of Springer Nature 2018   137
A. E. M. Eltorai et al. (eds.), *Essential Orthopedic Review*,
https://doi.org/10.1007/978-3-319-78387-1_62

(continued)

What is the eponym for the direct anterior approach to the hip?	Smith-Petersen
What is the eponym for the posterior approach to the hip?	Southern/Moore
What is the interval for the direct anterior approach to the hip?	Superficial: TFL/Sartorius Deep: Rectus femoris/gluteus medius
What is a major danger in the direct anterior approach to the hip?	Lateral femoral cutaneous nerve
What is a major danger in the direct posterior approach to the hip?	Sciatic nerve
What is the classic position of posterior hip dislocations?	Flexion, adduction, and internal rotation
What is the classic position for anterior dislocation of the hip?	Extension, abduction, and external rotation

Chapter 63
Osteonecrosis

Stephen Marcaccio

Define avascular necrosis.	An orthopedic phenomenon characterized by decreased vascular perfusion to the bones supporting the hip joint resulting in bone destruction and joint breakdown
List three direct causes of AVN.	1. Irradiation 2. Trauma 3. Hematologic disease (leukemia)
List three indirect causes of AVN.	1. Alcoholism 2. Hypercoaguable state 3. Chronic steroid use 4. Idiopathic

(continued)

S. Marcaccio, MD
Department of Orthopaedic Surgery, Rhode Island Hospital, Brown University, Providence, RI, USA
e-mail: stephen_marcaccio@brown.edu

© Springer International Publishing AG, part of Springer Nature 2018   139
A. E. M. Eltorai et al. (eds.), *Essential Orthopedic Review*,
https://doi.org/10.1007/978-3-319-78387-1_63

(continued)

What is the name of the classification system for AVN?	The Steinberg Classification (modified Ficat)
What is the most sensitive and specific imaging test for detecting AVN?	MRI
What is the most common method of conservative management for AVN?	Bisphosphonates
List three operative interventions for management of AVN.	1. Core decompression with bone grafting 2. Rotational osteotomy 3. Total hip resurfacing

Chapter 64
Total Hip Arthroplasty

Nicholas Lemme and Alexandre Boulos

What are the four most popular surgical approaches to the hip?	Posterior/posterolateral; direct lateral, anterolateral, direct anterior
What are the four components that make up a total hip arthroplasty?	1. Acetabular shell 2. Acetabular lining 3. Femoral head 4. Distal stem

(continued)

N. Lemme, MD (✉) · A. Boulos, MD
Department of Orthopaedics, Brown University, Providence, RI, USA
e-mail: nicholas_lemme@brown.edu; alexandre_boulos@brown.edu

© Springer International Publishing AG, part of Springer Nature 2018   141
A. E. M. Eltorai et al. (eds.), *Essential Orthopedic Review*,
https://doi.org/10.1007/978-3-319-78387-1_64

(continued)

What are the intervals for the posterior/posterolateral approach to the hip and what are the structures at risk?	Gluteus maximus (inferior gluteal nerve) and gluteus medius/tensor fascia lata (superior gluteal nerve) Structures at risk are sciatic nerve, inferior gluteal artery, and medial femoral circumflex artery
What are the superficial and deep intervals for the direct anterior approach to the hip and what are the structures at risk?	Superficial: Sartorius (femoral nerve) and tensor fasciae lata (superior gluteal nerve) Deep: Gluteus medius (superior gluteal nerve) and rectus femoris (femoral nerve) Structures at risk: Lateral femoral cutaneous nerve, ascending branch of lateral femoral circumflex
What is the recommended placement of the cup in the acetabulum?	30–50° Abduction and 5–25° anteversion
What are the two methods of prosthetic fixation for a THA?	1. Cement fixation (polymethylmethacrylate) 2. Bone in-growth fixation (porous)
What is the classification system used for post-op periprosthetic femur fractures?	Vancouver classification
What is the most common nerve injury seen in THA?	Peroneal branch of sciatic nerve, because it is closest to the acetabulum
What are the common causes of **intraoperative** periprosthetic femur fractures?	1. Placing a femoral component that is too large 2. Aggressive rasping during bone preparation 3. Rapid impaction of femoral component
What are risk factors for **post-operative** periprosthetic femur fractures?	1. Poor bone quality 2. Cementless prostheses 3. Compromised bone stock 4. History of revisions

What is the most common direction of hip dislocation following THA?	75–90% occur posteriorly
Which hip positions put one at most risk for a posterior dislocation following a posterior approach?	Hip flexion and internal rotation
Which hip positions put one at most risk for an anterior dislocation following an anterior approach?	Hip extension and external rotation
What are the surgical-related factors that increase the risk of dislocation following THA?	1. Soft tissue tension 2. Component position 3. Impingement 4. Head size 5. Acetabular lining profile
What can be done to prevent heterotopic ossification in a predisposed patient?	1 time dose of radiation or indomethacin
How can a periprosthetic femur fracture with an unstable implant be treated?	Replace implant with longer stem that passes the fracture site
Why is it important for a surgeon to replicate the offset when performing a THA?	1. Allows for balancing of soft tissue resulting in improved hip stability 2. Prevents leg length discrepancies
Which is the safest zone for the placement of acetabular screws and what neurovascular structures are at risk in this zone?	Posterior-superior zone Structures: superior gluteal nerve/vessels and the sciatic nerve

Chapter 65
Femoral Shaft Fractures

James Levins

When evaluating and treating a high-energy femoral shaft fracture, what other type of femur fracture in the ipsilateral leg must you have a high suspicion for?	Ipsilateral femoral neck fracture (up to 9% co-incidence with shaft fractures, obtain a CT scan with fine cuts through the femoral neck) [1]
What four aspects of the operative extremity do you need to check after fixing a femoral shaft fracture?	Length, rotation, femoral neck (for fracture), knee exam for ligamentous injury
How much blood can potentially be lost in the thigh from a femoral shaft fracture?	1–1.5 L

(continued)

J. Levins, MD
Orthopaedic Surgery, Brown University, Providence, RI, USA

© Springer International Publishing AG, part of Springer Nature 2018   145
A. E. M. Eltorai et al. (eds.), *Essential Orthopedic Review*,
https://doi.org/10.1007/978-3-319-78387-1_65

(continued)

In a mid-shaft femur fracture, what position does the proximal femoral segment usually rest relative to the distal segment, and why?	Varus—from the gluteal muscles and external rotators which abduct the proximal segment (the adductor mass will translate the distal segment medially) Flexed—from the psoas which flexes the proximal segment (the gastrocnemius inserts above knee on posterior femoral condyles and extends the distal segment relative to the proximal)
What two approaches may be used for intramedullary nailing of a femoral shaft fracture?	Anterograde (piriformis—or trochanteric-entry nail) or retrograde
Is there a difference in union rate between anterograde and retrograde nailing of a mid-shaft femur fracture?	No
If placing a tibial traction pin for a femur fracture, which side of the tibia should you start your incision and why?	Laterally, to avoid injury to the common peroneal nerve
In an unstable poly-traumatized patient who is taken emergently to the OR with neurosurgery for a closed head injury and noted to have a femoral shaft fracture, why would it be prudent to perform external fixation instead of intramedullary nailing?	To avoid further hypotension by minimizing time under anesthesia, limiting blood loss and lowering the risk of fat emboli, i.e., damage control orthopedics

Reference

1. Tornetta P, Kin MSH, Creevy WR. Diagnosis of femoral neck fractures in patients with a femoral shaft fracture. J Bone Joint Surg. 2007;89A:39–43.

Chapter 66
Ligamentous Knee Injury

James Levins

Classically, what injuries compose the "unhappy triad" or "terrible triad" injury to the knee?	Anterior cruciate ligament (ACL), medial collateral ligament (MCL), medial meniscus injury
Which meniscus (medial or lateral) is commonly injured in an acute ACL rupture?	Lateral meniscus
What is the reason for the limited healing potential of the cruciate ligaments relative to the collateral ligaments?	Intra-articular structures have poor blood supply relative to the rich extra-articular supply
What motion does the ACL primarily prevent?	Anterior tibial translation

(continued)

J. Levins, MD
Department of Orthopaedic Surgery, Brown University, Providence, RI, USA

© Springer International Publishing AG, part of Springer Nature 2018   147
A. E. M. Eltorai et al. (eds.), *Essential Orthopedic Review*,
https://doi.org/10.1007/978-3-319-78387-1_66

(continued)

What knee injury is commonly seen in a dashboard-type injury where a patient sustains a posterior acetabular wall fracture?	Posterior cruciate ligament (PCL) tear
When performing ACL reconstruction, what technical error is associated with early ACL failure?	Vertically oriented ACL graft, often resulting from a femoral tunnel placed too anteriorly
A patient has a multi-ligamentous knee injury after a motorcycle accident, suspicious for a knee dislocation that was reduced in the field. What studies would you want to obtain urgently?	Pulse exam, ankle-brachial index (ABI), CT angiogram if ABI <0.9 (due to the risk of popliteal artery injury)

Chapter 67
Meniscal Tear

Jonathan Hodax

What are the three zones of the meniscus?	Central: The "white-white," or avascular zone
	Middle: The "red-white," or partially vascularized zone
	Peripheral: The "red-red," or vascularized zone
What meniscus tears can be repaired?	Only those in the vascular zones of the meniscus (peripheral tears)
What is the "gold standard" technique for meniscal repair?	Vertical mattress sutures in an "inside out" technique (meaning the suture needle is passed from within the joint to outside the joint)

(continued)

J. Hodax, MD, MS
Department of Orthopedics, Rhode Island Hospital,
Providence, RI, USA

© Springer International Publishing AG, part of Springer Nature 2018   149
A. E. M. Eltorai et al. (eds.), *Essential Orthopedic Review*,
https://doi.org/10.1007/978-3-319-78387-1_67

(continued)

In what population is the medial meniscus more likely to be injured?	Older patients with degenerative tears
In what population is the lateral meniscus more likely to be injured?	Younger patients with an acute injury, especially together with an ACL tear
What is the effect of removing or debriding some or all of the meniscus?	Increased joint contact pressure, decreased joint stability, and an overall faster progression to arthritis

Chapter 68
Extensor Mechanism Injuries of the Knee

Jonathan Hodax

What are the components of the extensor mechanism?	The quadriceps, the quadriceps tendon, the patella, the patellar tendon, and the tibial tubercle
In what age group are each of the components of the extensor mechanism injured?	Tibial tubercle: Patients with open physes (pediatric patients)
	Patellar tendon: Patients <40 years old
	Patellar tendon: Patients <40 years old
	Quad tendon: Patients >40 years old
	Patellar fractures: Any age

(continued)

J. Hodax, MD, MS
Department of Orthopedics, Rhode Island Hospital,
Providence, RI, USA

© Springer International Publishing AG, part of Springer Nature 2018   151
A. E. M. Eltorai et al. (eds.), *Essential Orthopedic Review*,
https://doi.org/10.1007/978-3-319-78387-1_68

(continued)

What physical exam finding is an indication for operative management in suspected quad tendon rupture, patellar tendon rupture, or patellar fracture?	Inability to straight leg raise, or an "extensor lag" of 30°
What allows some patients with complete transverse patella fractures to still perform a straight leg raise?	An intact medial and lateral retinaculum
What kind of suture is typically used on the quad tendon and the patellar tendon to prevent suture cut-out?	A running locking stitch, typically a "Krackow"
What are the ways tendon can be repaired back to the patella?	Suture can be passed through bone tunnels and tied or can be fixed to the bone using suture anchors

Chapter 69
Lower Extremity Tibia and Fibula Shaft Fractures

Tyler S. Pidgeon

When treated with closed reduction, what are the acceptable parameters for angulation in the sagittal and coronal planes as well as rotation and length in tibia shaft fractures?	Less than 10° of flexion/extension and 5° of varus/valgus. There should be 50% cortical apposition, less than 1 cm of shortening, and less than 10° of rotational malalignment
Proximal third tibia shaft fractures classically fall into what deformity during intramedullary nailing?	Procurvatum (apex anterior) and valgus

(continued)

T. S. Pidgeon, MD
Department of Orthopaedic Surgery, The Warren Alpert Medical School at Brown University, Providence, RI, USA

© Springer International Publishing AG, part of Springer Nature 2018   153
A. E. M. Eltorai et al. (eds.), *Essential Orthopedic Review*,
https://doi.org/10.1007/978-3-319-78387-1_69

(continued)

To avoid deformity during intramedullary nailing of proximal third tibia shaft fractures, name three techniques that may be used.	Blocking screws (posterior and lateral to avoid procurvatum and valgus, respectively), unicortical plating, and semi-extended or suprapatellar approaches
What is the most common complication of intramedullary nailing of tibia shaft fractures?	Anterior knee pain (>50% of cases)
Describe the Gustilo-Anderson classification for open tibia fractures.	Type I: Wound <1 cm; minimal periosteal stripping. Type II: Wound 1–10 cm; mild to moderate periosteal stripping. Type III A: Wound >10 cm; substantial periosteal stripping and soft tissue injury; no flap required. Type III B: Substantial periosteal stripping and soft tissue injury; flap required due to inadequate soft tissue coverage. Type III C: Substantial soft tissue injury with vascular injury requiring repair
In open tibia fractures what is the most important intervention in reducing infection?	Early administration of antibiotics
According to the LEAP study, what is the most critical predictor for amputation in open tibia fractures?	Severity of soft tissue injury
In patients with tibia fractures, what is the most sensitive diagnostic test (other than physical exam) for the diagnosis of compartment syndrome?	Compartment pressure monitoring demonstrating a compartment pressure within 30 mmHg of the patient's pre-operative diastolic blood pressure

What are the advantages of intramedullary nailing compared to closed reduction and casting of tibia shaft fractures?	Decreased time to union and decreased time to weight bearing
How does the time to union compare between treatment of tibia shaft fractures with intramedullary nailing vs. plating?	Time to union is equivalent between these methods

Chapter 70
Distal Femoral Fractures

Viorel Raducan

What is the definition of a distal femoral fracture?	Fractures in the area 5 cm's proximal to the distal femoral joint line
What is the age distribution of distal femoral fractures?	Bimodal—young and elderly
What is the mechanism of injury of distal femoral fractures in the young population?	High energy trauma
What is the mechanism of injury in the elderly population?	Low energy trauma—fall from standing height
How are distal femoral fractures classified?	Extraarticular/intraarticular/periprosthetic

(continued)

V. Raducan, MD, FRCS(C)
Department of Orthopaedic Surgery, Marshall University School of Medicine, Huntington, WV, USA
e-mail: raducan@marshall.edu

© Springer International Publishing AG, part of Springer Nature 2018   157
A. E. M. Eltorai et al. (eds.), *Essential Orthopedic Review*,
https://doi.org/10.1007/978-3-319-78387-1_70

(continued)

What is the typical displacement of distal femoral fractures	Extension (gastrocnemius), shortening (hamstrings), and varum (adductors)
What structure is at risk in (displaced) distal femoral fractures and all injuries around the knee?	Popliteal artery—emphasis on vascular exam, presence of distal pulses
What is the imaging study of choice for fractures of the distal femur?	X-rays—knee (AP/lateral/obliques), full length femur
What is a Hoffa fracture?	Fracture of the lateral condyle of the femur in the coronal plane
What is the indication for CT scan in distal femur fractures?	Intraarticular extension, preoperative planning
What is the indication for angiography in distal femoral fractures?	Absence of distal pulses especially if no recovery after limb alignment (in line traction)
What is the preferred treatment for distal femoral fractures?	Surgery—open reduction and internal fixation
When can nonoperative treatment be considered in fractures of the distal femur?	Prohibitive surgical risk. Relative indication—non displaced fractures
What are the implants of choice for the surgical treatment of distal femoral fractures?	Fixed angle devices and retrograde intramedullary nails
What are the goals of surgery in distal femoral fractures?	Re-establish the anatomical knee axis and an anatomical joint line with stable internal fixation allowing early active range of motion
What are the complications after treatment of distal femoral fractures?	Malunion, varum nonunion (19%), and symptomatic hardware

Chapter 71
Patellar Fractures

Brian H. Cohen

What is the extensor mechanism of the knee made up of? What function does the extensor mechanism have?	Quadriceps muscle, quadriceps tendon, medial and lateral retinaculum, patellofemoral and patellotibial ligaments, patella, patellar tendon and tibial tubercle, extension of the knee
What are the two main facets of the patella? Which is larger? What is unique about the articular cartilage?	Lateral and medial facets, a vertical ridge divides the larger lateral facet (about 2/3 the area) from the smaller medial facet, the patella has the thickest articular cartilage in the body
What is the blood supply to the patella?	The geniculate arteries from an extraosseous arterial ring which also give the intraosseous blood supply

(continued)

B. H. Cohen, MD
Department of Orthopedic Surgery, Warren Alpert Medical School of Brown University, Providence, RI, USA

© Springer International Publishing AG, part of Springer Nature 2018   159
A. E. M. Eltorai et al. (eds.), *Essential Orthopedic Review*,
https://doi.org/10.1007/978-3-319-78387-1_71

(continued)

What is the mechanism of injury?	Usually, a direct blow or fall onto patella or indirect eccentric contraction, more common in patient <40 years old (Quadtriceps tendon tears more common in patients >40 years old)
What physical exam finding should you test? If intact what could be the reason for this?	Knee extension of the knee. Straight leg raise test. If able to extend knee, then the patellar retinaculum is intact
If there is a large hemarthrosis and it is difficult to exam patient due to pain what can you do?	Arthrocentesis with aspiration of the hemarthrosis and injection of lidocaine, then reexamine the knee for extension
What can be mistaken for a patella fracture on X-ray? What is it? Where is it most commonly located?	A bipartite patella which is a failure of ossification centers to fuse. It commonly bilateral (50%) and is located in the superior lateral quadrant of the patella
What are the types of patella fractures?	Transverse, pole (superior and inferior) or sleeve (inferior pole in childern), vertical, marginal, osteochondral, comminuted (stellate)
What are indications for nonoperative treatment? What is the treatment?	Intact extensor mechanism (able to straight leg raise), nondisplaced or minimally displaced fractures, vertical fracture, early weight bearing in extension in cylinder cast or locked hinged knee brace, begin early in range of motion in 2–3 weeks
What are surgical indications for patella fractures?	Open fractures, intraarticular step off of 2 mm or more, and the inability of the patient to extend knee actively
What are some surgical options of fixation?	Tension-band wiring, lag screw fixation, cerclage, cannulated lag screw with tension band, partial patellectomy, and total patellectomy

Chapter 72
Knee Tendon Rupture (Patellar and Quadriceps Tendons)

John R. Tuttle

What age and gender is most likely to be affected by patellar tendon rupture?	Males younger than 40
What exam finding would you expect with a complete patellar tendon rupture?	Loss of active knee extension or extensor lag
What radiographic findings might you expect and what imaging modality is the most sensitive to confirm the diagnosis?	Patella alta, MRI
What is the preferred treatment for acute, complete patellar tendon tears?	Primary repair

(continued)

J. R. Tuttle, MD, MS
Sports Medicine, Department of Orthopaedic Surgery, Virginia Tech Carilion School of Medicine, Roanoke, VA, USA
e-mail: jrtuttle@carilionclinic.org

© Springer International Publishing AG, part of Springer Nature 2018   161
A. E. M. Eltorai et al. (eds.), *Essential Orthopedic Review*,
https://doi.org/10.1007/978-3-319-78387-1_72

(continued)

What do you do if the tendon is not repairable?	Auto or allograft tendon reconstruction
What age and gender is more likely to be affected by quadriceps tendon rupture?	Males over 40
What are some risk factors for quad tendon rupture?	Renal failure, diabetes, RA, hyperparathyroidism, connective tissue disorders, steroids, cortisone injections
What radiographic finding would you expect with quad tendon rupture?	Patella baja
What is the preferred treatment for acute or chronic quad tendon rupture?	Primary repair, chronic injuries may require tendon lengthening (V-Y) or graft augmentation
What are some common complications following quad tendon repair?	Knee stiffness, strength deficit (nearly half of patients), inability to return to sports (about half of patients)

Bibliography

1. Brooks P. Extensor mechanism ruptures. Orthopedics. 2009;32(9).

Chapter 73
Patellar Dislocation

Steven F. DeFroda

What ligament is often injured in patellar dislocation?	Medial patellafemoral ligament (MPFL) [2]
What are risk factors for patellar dislocation? [1]	Hyperlaxity Trochlear dysplasia Lateral condyle hypoplasia High Q angle Prior instability event Excessive lateral patellar tilt Increased femoral anteversion Genu valgum External tibial torsion
What is "miserable malalignment syndrome"?	Combination of genu valgum, excessive femoral anteversion, and external tibial torsion. All contribute to high Q angle

(continued)

S. F. DeFroda, MD, ME
Department of Orthopaedic Surgery, Warren Alpert Medical School of Brown University, Providence, RI, USA

© Springer International Publishing AG, part of Springer Nature 2018   163
A. E. M. Eltorai et al. (eds.), *Essential Orthopedic Review*,
https://doi.org/10.1007/978-3-319-78387-1_73

(continued)

What type of bony injury is associated with patellar dislocation?	Avulsion fracture of medial patellar facet and/or impaction fracture of lateral femoral condyle [2]
What is the best way to assess patellar tilt?	Sunrise view radiograph
What is the TT-TG distance?	Distance between lines drawn perpendicular to posterior tibial cortex at the level of the tibial tubercle and trochlear groove on axial CT/MRI cuts
What is an abnormal TT-TG distance?	Greater than 15–20 mm

References

1. Khan N, Fithian D, Nomura E. In: Sanchis-Alfonso V, editor. Anterior knee pain and patellar Inestability. London: Springer; 2011. https://doi.org/10.1007/978-0-85729-507-1.
2. DeFroda SF, Hodax JD, Cruz AI. Patellar instability. J Pediatr. 2016;173:258–258.e1. https://doi.org/10.1016/j.jpeds.2016.03.025.
3. Waterman BR, Belmont PJ, Owens BD. Patellar dislocation in the United States: role of sex, age, race, and athletic participation. J Knee Surg. http://www.ncbi.nlm.nih.gov/pubmed/22624248. Published 2012. Accessed 27 Nov. 2015.
4. Fithian DC. Epidemiology and natural history of acute patellar dislocation. Am J Sports Med. 2004;32(5):1114–21. https://doi.org/10.1177/0363546503260788.
5. Chotel F, Bérard J, Raux S. Patellar instability in children and adolescents. Orthop Traumatol Surg Res. 2014;100(1 S):S125–37. https://doi.org/10.1016/j.otsr.2013.06.014.

Chapter 74
Total Knee Arthroplasty

Alexandre Boulos and Nicholas Lemme

Describe the X-ray findings of an arthritic knee	1. Joint space narrowing 2. Osteophytes 3. Subchondral sclerosis 4. Subchondral cyst
What is the difference between the anatomic and mechanical axis of the femur?	The anatomic axis runs from the top of the greater trochanter straight through the center of the femur and down to the middle of the ankle. The mechanical axis extends from the center of the femoral head through the medial tibial spine and down to the center of the ankle joint

(continued)

A. Boulos, MD (✉) · N. Lemme, MD
Department of Orthopedics, Brown University,
Providence, RI, USA
e-mail: nicholas_lemme@brown.edu;
alexandre_boulos@brown.edu

© Springer International Publishing AG, part of Springer Nature 2018   165
A. E. M. Eltorai et al. (eds.), *Essential Orthopedic Review*,
https://doi.org/10.1007/978-3-319-78387-1_74

(continued)

What is the normal position of the anatomic axis relative to the mechanical axis? How do those change in osteoarthritis?	The anatomic axis is normally 6° of valgus from the mechanical axis. In most people with OA, this angle will be in relative varus
What are the most common approaches for simple primary TKA?	1. Medial parapatellar approach 2. Midvastus 3.Subvastus 4. Minimally invasive
What is the interval for the medial parapatellar approach to the knee?	The interval lies between the rectus femoris muscle and the vastus medialis
What structure can be identified in the posterior aspect of the lateral compartment of the knee?	The popliteus muscle
Which structure is responsible for blood supply to the patella after TKA with a medial approach?	Superior lateral genicular artery
What are the two most commonly used techniques for balancing the flexion and extension gaps during TKA?	1. Measured resection 2. Gap balancing (soft-tissue tension balancing)
What is the preferred rotation of the femoral and tibial components and why?	External rotation of the femoral and tibial components decreases the Q angle and the strain on the lateral retinaculum. This helps to prevent patella maltracking and dislocation postoperatively

What are the five most common causes of failure in TKA?	1. Aseptic loosening—MCC after 2 years 2. Septic failure—MCC within 2 years 3. Ligamentous instability/flexor mechanism disruption 4. Periprosthetic fracture 5. Arthrofibrosis
How do the following affect the flexion/extension gaps, respectively: 　1. Changing the distal femur? 　2. Changing the femoral component size? 　3. Changing the proximal tibia or changing the polyethylene insert?	1. Changing the distal femur will only change the extension gap 2. Changing the femoral component size will only change the flexion gap 3. Any chance to the proximal tibia or the insert will change both the extension and flexion gaps
What neurovascular structures should be assessed after TKA?	1. Check DP and PT pulse 2. Check function of deep and superficial peroneal nerves
What are risk factors for periprosthetic fractures after TKA?	1. Poor bone quality 2. Mechanical stress-risers 3. Neurological disorders
What classification system is used for periprosthetic fractures of the knee?	Lewis and Rorabeck for distal femur fractures Felix for tibial fractures
A patient with history of TKA presents with knee pain and instability. What studies should you order?	1. CBC, ESR, CRP, knee aspiration with cell count and culture 2. X-rays of the joint

(continued)

(continued)

What is the difference between a constrained and unconstrained implant?	Prosthetics used in TKA can be broadly classified as constrained or unconstrained Constraint refers the valgus and varus stability provided by the implant. An unconstrained implant does not offer this stability and instead relies on the native MCL and LCL for this function
What are the two types of constrained implants and what are the differences?	Constrained implants can either be hinged or unhinged. The hinge refers to an axle connecting the tibial and femoral components. A nonhinged design may be used for isolated LCL or MCL instability while a hinged design is preferred for global ligamentous instability or hyperextension instability
What are the two types of unconstrained implants?	Cruciate retaining and posterior stabilizing
What is a cruciate retaining implant and what are the indications for its use? What are pros and cons?	Cruciate retaining implants rely on an intact PCL for posterior stabilization. They are usually used for patients with stable knees and no significant valgus or varus deformities. Patients have improved proprioception and do not experience impingement. However, a rupture PCL may lead to instability and a need for revision
What is a posterior stabilizing implant and what are the indications for its use? What are pros and cons?	Posterior stabilizing implants have a constraint that provides the stability of the PCL, which is removed during surgery. It is preferred some patients with inflammatory arthritis. Patients have better ROM and no risk of PCL rupture. Disadvantages include the possibility of impingement, dislocation, and patellar clunk syndrome

Chapter 75
Patellofemoral Pain Syndrome

Steven F. DeFroda

What is the purpose of the patella?	Acts as a fulcrum to transmit forces across the knee
How much force does the patellofemoral joint experience?	Approximately 5–10 times body weight
What is the first-line management of patellofemoral syndrome?	Symptomatic management with NSAIDs, muscle strengthening around the knee, and weight loss
What is the typical pathology involved?	Chondromalacia of the patellofemoral joint
What is the outerbridge classification of chondromalacia?	Type 1: softening Type 2: fissuring Type 3: crabmeat changes with no subchondral bone exposed Type 4: subchondral bone exposed

S. F. DeFroda, MD, ME
Department of Orthopaedic Surgery, Warren Alpert Medical School of Brown University, Providence, RI, USA

© Springer International Publishing AG, part of Springer Nature 2018   169
A. E. M. Eltorai et al. (eds.), *Essential Orthopedic Review*,
https://doi.org/10.1007/978-3-319-78387-1_75

Reference

1. Crossley KM, Callaghan MJ, van Linschoten R. Patellofemoral pain. BMJ. 2015;351:h3939. http://www.ncbi.nlm.nih.gov/pubmed/26537829. Accessed 9 May 2017.

Chapter 76
IT Band Syndrome

John R. Tuttle

What anatomic structures are involved in IT band syndrome and where does it hurt?	IT band rubbing over lateral femoral condyle, pain is over lateral femoral condyle
What limb alignment issue is associated with IT band syndrome?	Genu varum or recurvatum
What is the origin, insertion, and innervation of the IT band?	Continuation of tensor fascia lata, Gerdy's tubercle, superior gluteal nerve (L1–3)
What is the main treatment method?	IT band stretching
Do the majority of patients improve without surgery?	Yes
What surgical intervention is appropriate if nonoperative treatment fails?	IT band windowing over lateral femoral epicondyle, IT band lengthening in refractory cases

J. R. Tuttle, MD, MS
Sports Medicine, Department of Orthopaedic Surgery, Virginia Tech Carilion School of Medicine, Roanoke, VA, USA
e-mail: jrtuttle@carilionclinic.org

© Springer International Publishing AG, part of Springer Nature 2018   171
A. E. M. Eltorai et al. (eds.), *Essential Orthopedic Review*,
https://doi.org/10.1007/978-3-319-78387-1_76

Bibliography

1. Beals C, Flanigan D. A review of treatments for iliotibial band syndrome in the athletic population. J Sports Med. 2013;2013:367169. https://doi.org/10.1155/2013/367169.

Chapter 77
Lower Extremity Tibial Plateau Fractures

Tyler S. Pidgeon

Recite the Schatzker classification for tibial plateau fractures	Type I: Lateral Split; Type II: Lateral Split/Depressed; Type III: Lateral Depressed; Type IV: Medial; Type V: Bicondylar; Type VI: Metaphysis/Diaphysis Dissociation
What severe knee injury is a medial tibial plateau fracture said to be equivalent to?	Knee dislocation
What test helps to rule out a vascular injury in a patient with a tibial plateau fracture?	Ankle-Brachial Index (ABI). ABI of <0.9 has high sensitivity and specificity for diagnosis of a vascular injury and warrants further workup

(continued)

T. S. Pidgeon, MD
Department of Orthopaedic Surgery, The Warren Alpert Medical School at Brown University, Providence, RI, USA

© Springer International Publishing AG, part of Springer Nature 2018   173
A. E. M. Eltorai et al. (eds.), *Essential Orthopedic Review*,
https://doi.org/10.1007/978-3-319-78387-1_77

(continued)

After ORIF of tibial plateau fractures what is the best indicator of long-term outcomes?	Joint alignment and stability
What *temporizing* measure is indicated in a patient with a severely displaced tibial plateau fracture with substantial shortening, angulation, and/or impaction?	Knee-spanning external fixation
Patients with tibial plateau fractures are at risk for development of what condition considered to be an orthopedic emergency?	Compartment syndrome
What imaging modality is most useful in preoperative planning for tibial plateau fractures?	CT scan
Which meniscus is most commonly torn in patients with tibial plateau fractures?	Lateral meniscus
Bicondylar tibial plateau fractures undergoing ORIF should be considered for what type of fixation?	Lateral and medial plating
Describe the shape and position of the lateral and medial tibial plateau	Lateral: Convex and proximal; Medial: Concave and distal

Chapter 78
Stress Fracture

John R. Tuttle

When overuse results in trabecular microfractures from repetitive pressure applied to a *normal* bone, it is called what?	Fatigue fracture (a subtype of stress fracture)
When overuse results in trabecular microfractures from repetitive pressure applied to an *abnormal* bone, it is called what?	Insufficiency fracture (a subtype of stress fracture)
Stress fracture pain increases with ____ and improves with ____	Activity, rest
What is the most sensitive and specific diagnostic test for stress fractures?	MRI

(continued)

J. R. Tuttle, MD, MS
Sports Medicine, Department of Orthopaedic Surgery, Virginia Tech Carilion School of Medicine, Roanoke, VA, USA
e-mail: jrtuttle@carilionclinic.org

© Springer International Publishing AG, part of Springer Nature 2018   175
A. E. M. Eltorai et al. (eds.), *Essential Orthopedic Review*,
https://doi.org/10.1007/978-3-319-78387-1_78

(continued)

Should all stress fractures be treated without surgery, at least at first?	No (e.g., tension-sided femoral neck)
What athlete is at higher risk for stress fractures in ribs 4–9?	Rowers
Bisphosphonate medication has been linked to what anatomic site of stress fracture?	Subtrochanteric femur fracture
What three conditions must you address in a female athlete with a stress fracture?	Amenorrhea, eating disorder, osteoporosis (female triad)
What is the most common lower extremity stress fracture site and how common is it among all stress fractures?	Tibia, accounts for half of all stress fractures
What is the second most common site for stress fractures and which populations tend to be affected by them?	Metatarsals (most common: second and third), military recruits (marching), and ballet dancers (en pointe)

Bibliography

1. Astur DC, Zanatta F, Arliani GG, Moraes ER, Pochini A de C, Ejnisman B. Stress fractures: definition, diagnosis and treatment. Rev Bras Ortop. 2016;51(1):3–10. https://doi.org/10.1016/j.rboe.2015.12.008.

Chapter 79
Metatarsalgia

Stephen Marcaccio

Define metatarsalgia.	Symptom of pain experienced in the ball of the foot
List three causes of metatarsalgia.	Traumatic (MTP dislocations) Acquired (hallux valgus) Infectious (synovitis/osteomyelitis)
Define Morton's neuroma.	Compressive neuropathy of the interdigital nerve
Where is Morton's neuroma most commonly located?	Commonly involves the second/third interdigital nerve between the metatarsal heads

(continued)

S. Marcaccio, MD
Department of Orthopaedic Surgery, Rhode Island Hospital, Brown University, Providence, RI, USA
e-mail: stephen_marcaccio@brown.edu

© Springer International Publishing AG, part of Springer Nature 2018   177
A. E. M. Eltorai et al. (eds.), *Essential Orthopedic Review*,
https://doi.org/10.1007/978-3-319-78387-1_79

(continued)

What physical exam findings are common with Morton's neuroma?	Positive web space compression test Mulder's click (felt when squeezing metatarsals together)
What is the technique for operative management of Morton's neuroma?	Cut the interdigital nerve as far proximal as possible to prevent recurrence
Which metatarsal is the most common involved with stress fractures?	The second metatarsal
What is the best radiographic method to detect? Acute osteomyelitis or chronic?	Acute: MRI Chronic: X-ray

Chapter 80
Hallux Valgus

Rishin J. Kadakia and Jason T. Bariteau

Hallux Valgus Questions and Answers	
What is another common name for hallux valgus?	Bunion deformity
What two types of hallux valgus exist?	Adult and juvenile
How do you describe the great toe in hallux valgus?	Hallux is in valgus and pronated
What symptoms are common with hallux valgus	Pain over medial prominence with shoe wear, pain with range of motion of first toe
What is the first-line treatment for hallux valgus?	Shoe modification (wide toe box shoe), toe spacers, and orthotics

(continued)

R. J. Kadakia, MD (✉) · J. T. Bariteau, MD
Department of Orthopaedic Surgery, Emory University School of Medicine, Atlanta, GA, USA
e-mail: rishin.j.kadakia@emory.edu

© Springer International Publishing AG, part of Springer Nature 2018   179
A. E. M. Eltorai et al. (eds.), *Essential Orthopedic Review*,
https://doi.org/10.1007/978-3-319-78387-1_80

(continued)

Hallux Valgus Questions and Answers	
What are some differences between adult hallux valgus and juvenile hallux valgus?	Juvenile hallux valgus is often bilateral, familial, usually not painful (more cosmetic concerns)
The sesamoids are found within which muscle's tendons?	Flexor hallucis brevis
What is the hallux valgus angle (HVA)?	Angle between a line through the long axis of the first metatarsal and a ling through the long axis of the proximal phalanx
What is the intermetatarsal angle (IMA)?	Angle between the long axis of the first metatarsal and the second metatarsal
What is considered normal for the HVA?	Less than or equal to 15°
What is considered normal for the IMA?	Less than or equal to 9°
What are the names of some of the distally based osteotomies of the first metatarsal commonly used in correction of hallux valgus?	Chevron, Mitchell
What are the names of the proximally based osteotomies of the first metatarsal commonly used in correction of hallux valgus?	Scarf, Ludloff
What is the indication for a Lapidus procedure?	First TMTJ instability, Lapidis is a fusion of the first TMTJ

Chapter 81
Heel Pain

Stephen Marcaccio

What significant anatomical tendons/nerves are located around the heel?	Achilles tendon, foot/toe flexor bundle, tibial neurovascular bundle, plantar fascia
From a lateral view, what is the anatomic relationship of the tibialis posterior, FDL, and FHL?	Anterior to posterior: tibialis posterior, FDL, nerve, then HFL ("Tom, Dick, and Nervous Harry")
What are the differences in outcomes between operative and nonoperative management of Achilles tendon ruptures?	Studies have shown that there are minimal long-term differences between the two methods of management
What is the name of the stitch used for Achilles tendon repair?	The Krackow stitch
What is the most common type of tarsal fracture?	Calcaneus fracture

(continued)

S. Marcaccio, MD
Department of Orthopaedic Surgery, Rhode Island Hospital, Brown University, Providence, RI, USA
e-mail: stephen_marcaccio@brown.edu

© Springer International Publishing AG, part of Springer Nature 2018
A. E. M. Eltorai et al. (eds.), *Essential Orthopedic Review*,
https://doi.org/10.1007/978-3-319-78387-1_81

(continued)

What are the names of the two classification systems for intra-articular calcaneus fractures?	The Essex-Lopresti and sanders classification systems
What is a normal Bohler angle measurement?	40°
What is a normal angle of Gissane?	130–145°
What is the value of MRI in the diagnosis of calcaneus fractures?	Can be used to diagnose calcaneal stress fractures in the presence of normal radiographs or uncertain diagnosis

Chapter 82
Ankle Sprain/Fracture

Rishin J. Kadakia and Jason T. Bariteau

What defines a high ankle sprain?	Syndesmotic injury
What ligament is most commonly damaged in ankle sprains	Anterior talofibular ligament (ATFL)
What are the three lateral ligaments of the ankle joint?	Anterior talofibular ligament (ATFL), calcaneofibular ligament (CFL), posterior talofibular ligament (PFL)
What are common associated injuries seen in patients with ankle sprains	Osteochondral fractures/defects, peroneal tendon pathology

(continued)

R. J. Kadakia, MD (✉) · J. T. Bariteau, MD
Department of Orthopaedic Surgery, Emory University School of Medicine, Atlanta, GA, USA
e-mail: rishin.j.kadakia@emory.edu

© Springer International Publishing AG, part of Springer Nature 2018   183
A. E. M. Eltorai et al. (eds.), *Essential Orthopedic Review*,
https://doi.org/10.1007/978-3-319-78387-1_82

(continued)

What radiograph view can be used to identify a syndesmotic injury?	External rotation stress view
What is the normal measurement for the medial clear space?	Less than or equal to 4 mm
What is the normal measurement for the tibiofibular clear space?	Less than or equal to 6 mm
What imaging modality when evaluated for tendon pathology or osteochondral defects	MRI
What are the indications for surgery for ankle sprains	Persistent pain and/or instability after a long period of nonoperative treatment
What is the name of the procedure involving anatomic reconstruction of the lateral ankle ligaments?	Brostrom procedure/modified Brostrom procedure
What is name of one classification system for ankle fractures?	Lauge-Hansen
What is the most common type of ankle fracture based on the Lauge-Hansen system?	Supination external rotation

Chapter 83
Talar Fracture

Gregory R. Waryasz

What is the mechanism of a talar neck fracture?	Forced dorsiflexion with axial load
What does the lateral process of the talus articulate with?	Posterior facet of calcaneus and lateral malleolus of fibula
What Hawkins classification has the highest risk of AVN?	Hawkins IV
What is a Canale view?	Optimal view of talar neck. Maximum equinus, 15° pronation, and X-ray 75° cephalad from horizontal
What should be done with an extruded talus?	Clean, reduce, and ORIF

(continued)

G. R. Waryasz, MD, CSCS
Department of Orthopaedic Surgery, Massachusetts General Hospital, Boston, MA, USA

© Springer International Publishing AG, part of Springer Nature 2018   185
A. E. M. Eltorai et al. (eds.), *Essential Orthopedic Review*,
https://doi.org/10.1007/978-3-319-78387-1_83

(continued)

What is a Hawkins sign?	Subchondral lucency seen on mortise X-ray at 6–8 weeks representing intact vascularity and resorption of subchondral bone
What does a varus talar malunion lead to?	Decreased subtalar eversion and weightbearing on the lateral border of foot

Chapter 84
Calcaneus Fracture

Rishin J. Kadakia and Jason T. Bariteau

What is the most commonly fractured bone in the foot?	The calcaneus
What is the most common mechanism of injury that causes calcaneus fractures?	Axial loading of the foot
The calcaneus articulates with which other bones?	Talus and cuboid
How many facets are located on the superior articular surface of the calcaneus?	Three
The middle facet is located on the sustentaculum tali of the calcaneus, which tendon passes below this structure?	Flexor hallucis longus

(continued)

R. J. Kadakia, MD (✉) · J. T. Bariteau, MD
Department of Orthopaedic Surgery, Emory University School of Medicine, Atlanta, GA, USA
e-mail: rishin.j.kadakia@emory.edu

© Springer International Publishing AG, part of Springer Nature 2018   187
A. E. M. Eltorai et al. (eds.), *Essential Orthopedic Review*,
https://doi.org/10.1007/978-3-319-78387-1_84

(continued)

What angles obtained on a lateral radiograph of the calcaneus are used to evaluate calcaneus fractures?	Angle of Gissane and Bohler's angle
What other part of the body must be imaged in patients with calcaneus fractures?	Lumbar spine (high incidence of vertebral injuries)
Which classification system for calcaneus fractures requires CT scans and examines the articular fragments on coronal cuts?	Sanders classification
What radiographic view is typically obtained for calcaneus fractures that allows for visualization of the tuberosity and fracture alignment (varus/valgus)?	Harris view
What is the most common deformity seen with calcaneus fractures?	Lateral wall blow out with varus deformity and shortening of the calcaneus
Which facet of the subtalar joint is most commonly fractured with intra-articular calcaneus fractures?	The posterior facet

Chapter 85
Lisfranc Fracture

Gregory R. Waryasz

What is the mechanism of a Lisfranc fracture?	Hyperflexion/compression/abduction moment on forefoot and transmitted to the TMT articulation
What are the articulations of the Lisfrac joint complex?	Tarsometatarsal, intermetatarsal, intertarsal
What the Lisfranc ligament connect?	Medial cuneiform to base of second metatarsal on plantar surface
Where is the bruising usually present with a Lisfranc?	Plantar ecchymosis sign
What is the indication for ORIF with Lisfranc injury?	Greater than 2 mm displacement at the Lisfranc articulation

(continued)

G. R. Waryasz, MD, CSCS
Department of Orthopaedic Surgery, Massachusetts General Hospital, Boston, MA, USA

© Springer International Publishing AG, part of Springer Nature 2018   189
A. E. M. Eltorai et al. (eds.), *Essential Orthopedic Review*,
https://doi.org/10.1007/978-3-319-78387-1_85

(continued)

What position do you place the foot in to stress the Lisfranc Ligament?	Passive abduction and pronation of the forefoot with a fixed hindfoot

Chapter 86
Metatarsal Fracture

Seth W. O'Donnell and Brad D. Blankenhorn

Where is the most common location of metatarsal (MT) stress fractures?	Second MT
What injury must be looked for with multiple proximal MT fractures?	Lisfranc/Lisfranc equivalent injuries
Do MT fractures need surgery?	Most heal with conservative treatment
What medical workup should occur in females with MT stress fractures?	Metabolic bone disease/amenorrhea
What is the primary nonoperative treatment?	Stiff soled shoe or CAM walker boot

(continued)

S. W. O'Donnell, MD (✉) · B. D. Blankenhorn, MD
Department of Orthopaedic Surgery, Warren Alpert Medical School of Brown University, Providence, RI, USA

© Springer International Publishing AG, part of Springer Nature 2018   191
A. E. M. Eltorai et al. (eds.), *Essential Orthopedic Review*,
https://doi.org/10.1007/978-3-319-78387-1_86

(continued)

What is a Jones fracture?	Fracture of the fifth MT base in the "watershed" region of poor bone healing/often involving the MT—cuboid articulation
What is a dancer's fracture?	Fracture of the fifth MT shaft
How long should patients remain non-weightbearing?	Most MT fractures can bear immediate weight as tolerated

Chapter 87
Pilon Fracture

Seth W. O'Donnell and Brad D. Blankenhorn

Define a pilon fracture	Fracture of tibial plafond, involves articular surface of distal tibia, often from a high energy axial load
What is the chaput fragment?	Fragment attached to anterior inferior tibiofibular ligament, anterolateral aspect of distal tibia
What initial treatment is often used?	External fixation
What advanced imaging can be used to gather more information about the fracture?	CT scan (obtain *after* reduction and external fixation)

(continued)

S. W. O'Donnell (✉) · B. D. Blankenhorn, MD
Department of Orthopaedic Surgery, Warren Alpert Medical School of Brown University, Providence, RI, USA

© Springer International Publishing AG, part of Springer Nature 2018   193
A. E. M. Eltorai et al. (eds.), *Essential Orthopedic Review*,
https://doi.org/10.1007/978-3-319-78387-1_87

(continued)

What is a common risk factor for wound or bone healing issues?	Smoking
What structure is the posterior inferior tibiofibular ligament attached to?	Volkmann fragment of the distal tibia
What is the fibular attachment of the anterior inferior tibiofibular ligament called?	Wagstaff fragment

Chapter 88
Achilles Tendon Pathology

Gregory R. Waryasz

Where does an Achilles rupture usually occur?	4–6 cm above calaneal insertion in the hypovascular area
What antibiotic class is associated with Achilles ruptures?	Fluoroquinolones
What is a Thompson test?	Lack of plantarflexion when the calf is squeezed
What is the tendon can be transferred in chronic Achilles rupture cases?	Flexor hallucis longus
What nerve is directly lateral to the Achilles tendon?	Sural
What are some risk factors to wound healing complications following Achilles repair?	Smoking, females, steroid use, open technique

(continued)

G. R. Waryasz, MD, CSCS
Department of Orthopaedic Surgery, Massachusetts General Hospital, Boston, MA, USA

© Springer International Publishing AG, part of Springer Nature 2018   195
A. E. M. Eltorai et al. (eds.), *Essential Orthopedic Review*,
https://doi.org/10.1007/978-3-319-78387-1_88

(continued)

| What is the first line of treatment for insertional Achilles tendinopathy? | Activity modification, shoe wear modification, physical therapy |
| What is the histology of insertional Achilles tendinopathy? | Disorganized collagen with mucoid degeneration. Few inflammatory cells. Sometimes calcium deposits |

Chapter 89
Diabetic Foot

Seth W. O'Donnell and Brad D. Blankenhorn

What is the most etiology of diabetic foot ulcers?	Peripheral neuropathy
What test is more sensitive than light touch or two-point discrimination for determining loss of protective sensation?	Semmes-Weinstein 5.07 monofilament
What are some radiographic findings of Charcot foot?	Osteopenia, sclerosis, fragmentation, joint collapse, and destruction
What ABI is needed to ensure adequate vascular health for healing?	30–40 mmHg in toes and >70 mmHg at the ankle

(continued)

S. W. O'Donnell, MD (✉) · B. D. Blankenhorn, MD
Department of Orthopaedic Surgery, Warren Alpert Medical School of Brown University, Providence, RI, USA

© Springer International Publishing AG, part of Springer Nature 2018   197
A. E. M. Eltorai et al. (eds.), *Essential Orthopedic Review*,
https://doi.org/10.1007/978-3-319-78387-1_89

(continued)

What classification system is used to grade ulcers?	Wagner: 0—At risk, skin intact; 1—Superficial; 2—Deep without infection; 3—Deep infection; 4—Gangrene distal to midfoot; 5—Proximal gangrene
What are the most common infectious organisms?	Staph and strep species
Why should anaerobic antibiotic coverage be considered?	1/3 of infected diabetic feet have positive anaerobic cultures
What is the primary treatment when no infection is present?	Total contact casting, frequent re-evaluation and skin checks

Chapter 90
Charcot Arthropathy

Rishin J. Kadakia and Jason T. Bariteau

Define charcot arthropathy?	Progressive disorder involving destruction of bones and joints due to loss of protective sensation
What is the most common cause of charcot arthropathy in the foot and ankle?	Diabetes
What other joints are commonly affected by charcot arthropathy?	Knee, shoulder, elbow
What are the symptoms of charcot arthropathy in the foot and ankle?	Swelling, warmth, erythema, not always painful

(continued)

R. J. Kadakia, MD (✉) · J. T. Bariteau, MD
Department of Orthopaedic Surgery, Emory University School
of Medicine, Atlanta, GA, USA
e-mail: rishin.j.kadakia@emory.edu

© Springer International Publishing AG, part of Springer Nature 2018   199
A. E. M. Eltorai et al. (eds.), *Essential Orthopedic Review*,
https://doi.org/10.1007/978-3-319-78387-1_90

(continued)

How can you differentiate infection from charcot arthropathy in the foot and ankle?	Erythema will decrease when the extremity is elevated in charcot arthropathy
What test is used commonly used to diagnose diabetic neuropathy in charcot?	Semmes-Weinstein monofilament testing
What is the first line treatment for charcot arthropathy in the foot and ankle?	Total contact casting following by a CROW boot
What inflammatory markers are elevated in charcot arthropathy?	ESR and WBC
Why is deformity correction or arthrodesis not the best treatment strategy?	High complication rates with operative intervention
What are the temporal stages for progression of charcot arthropathy?	Fragmentation, coalescence, reconstruction
What is the name of the anatomic classification system for charcot arthropathy?	Brodsky classification

Chapter 91
Tarsal Tunnel Syndrome

Brian H. Cohen

What is the tarsal tunnel? What are the borders of the tarsal tunnel?	A fibroosseous tunnel located at the posteromedial ankle and hindfoot, the flexor retinaculum is roof and extends from the medial malleolus to the medial side of the calcaneal tuberosity. The medial distal tibia, talus, and calcaneus make up the floor
What is the content of the tarsal tunnel in order from medial to posterior? What is a mnemonic to remember?	Posterior tibial tendon, flexor digitorum longus tendon, posterior tibial artery and veins, tibial nerve and flexor hallucis longus tendon, (mnemonic to help remember order: Tom Dick and a Very Nervous Harry)

(continued)

B. H. Cohen MD
Department of Orthopedic Surgery, Warren Alpert Medical School
of Brown University, Providence, RI, USA

© Springer International Publishing AG, part of Springer Nature 2018   201
A. E. M. Eltorai et al. (eds.), *Essential Orthopedic Review*,
https://doi.org/10.1007/978-3-319-78387-1_91

(continued)

When dissecting on the medial side of ankle which muscle has the most distal muscle belly?	Flexor hallucis longus
What are the three terminal branches of the tibial nerve? Where do they branch? Which branches first?	Medial calcaneal nerve, lateral plantar nerve, and medial plantar nerve, within the tarsal tunnel just proximal and deep to the superior edge of the abductor hallucis muscle, the medial calcaneal nerve branches first
What is tarsal tunnel syndrome?	Tibial nerve entrapment beneath the flexor retinaculum or tarsal canal
What are some causes of tarsal tunnel syndrome?	Bone from prior distal tibial, talar, or calcaneal fractures, tenosynovitis, ganglia/cysts from a tendon sheath or subtalar/tibiotalar joints, bone and soft tissue from rheumatoid arthritis or ankylosing spondylitis, varicosities, neural tumor, tarsal coalition, and fixed valgus hindfoot which can cause a chronic traction neuropathy
What are some clinical findings of tarsal tunnel syndrome?	Dysthesias in the plantar aspect of the foot, toes, or medial distal calf
What are the two types of provocative test?	(1) Triple compression test—ankle is plantar flexed and the foot is inverted, then digital compression is applied over the tibial nerve (2) Dorsiflexion-eversion test—maximally evert the foot and dorsiflex the ankle passively, with all the metatarsophalangeal joints maximally dorsiflexed, hold position is held for 5–10 s

(continued)

What test should you order?	MRI, as most cases are caused by a space-occupying lesions
	Electrodiagnostic testing can be normal in patients with tarsal tunnel syndrome, helps rule out systemic neuropathies, a negative electrodiagnostic testing is not a contraindication for surgery
What are some conservative treatment options?	6–12 weeks of ankle immobilization in a night splint, anti-inflammatory agents, and shoe modification or orthosis, be careful with corticosteroid injections in this area as concern for tendon attenuation or rupture
What are the surgical options? Which patients do better?	Surgical decompression of tibial nerve. Patients with space-occupying lesions respond better to surgical decompression than those with idiopathic or traumatic causes, if no identifiable cause relief of symptoms is not predictable

Chapter 92
Peroneal Tendon Pathology

Seth W. O'Donnell and Brad D. Blankenhorn

Where do peroneal tendons cause pain?	Posterior lateral ankle
What structure is often damaged when peroneal tendons dislocate?	Superior peroneal retinaculum (SPR)
What provocative test can identify peroneal pathology?	Pain and tenderness in the posterior-lateral ankle which increases with resisted eversion
If symmetric weakness to eversion testing is present, what additional pathology should be considered?	Charcot-Marie-Tooth
What X-ray finding can suggest instability of the peroneal tendons?	"Fleck sign"—an avulsion of the distal fibular insertion of the SPR

(continued)

S. W. O'Donnell, MD (✉) · B. D. Blankenhorn, MD
Department of Orthopaedic Surgery, Warren Alpert Medical School of Brown University, Providence, RI, USA

© Springer International Publishing AG, part of Springer Nature 2018   205
A. E. M. Eltorai et al. (eds.), *Essential Orthopedic Review*,
https://doi.org/10.1007/978-3-319-78387-1_92

(continued)

What is the orientation of the tendons behind the fibula?	Peroneus brevis is anterior to peroneus longus
What is the common mechanism of peroneal injury?	Forced inversion of a plantar flexed foot
What imaging study can be helpful for dynamic information about the tendons?	Ultrasound
What imaging study is the gold standard for tendon/soft tissue pathology?	MRI

Chapter 93
Flatfoot

Seth W. O'Donnell and Brad D. Blankenhorn

What musculo-tendinous structure is often found to be insufficient?	Posterior tibial
What is another term for the superiomedial calcaneonavicular ligament?	Spring ligament
In children with recurrent ankle sprains or rigid flatfoot, what pathology should be evaluated?	Tarsal coalition
What muscle antagonizes the posterior tibialis?	Peroneus brevis
What is the major difference between Stage II and Stage III flatfoot deformity?	Flexible deformity (Stage II) vs. Rigid deformity (Stage III)

(continued)

S. W. O'Donnell, MD (✉) · B. D. Blankenhorn, MD
Department of Orthopaedic Surgery, Warren Alpert Medical
School of Brown University, Providence, RI, USA

© Springer International Publishing AG, part of Springer Nature 2018   207
A. E. M. Eltorai et al. (eds.), *Essential Orthopedic Review*,
https://doi.org/10.1007/978-3-319-78387-1_93

(continued)

Why can patients hurt on the outside of their ankle in severe disease?	Subfibular impingment
What is the too many toes sign?	An indicator of forefoot abduction, usually seen in Stage IIb disease

Chapter 94
Plantar Fasciitis

Gregory R. Waryasz

What are risk factors for plantar fasciitis?	Obesity, decreased ankle dorsiflexion, weight bearing endurance activities (dancing and running)
What are the symptoms of plantar fasciitis?	Insidious onset of heel pain, often first steps of day
Where is the patient usually most tender with plantar fasciitis?	Medial tuberosity of calcaneus/origin of the plantar fascia medially
What is Baxter's nerve?	First branch of lateral plantar nerve that can lead to heel pain around the origin of the abductor hallucis
What is the first line of treatment for plantar fasciitis?	Pain control, splinting, stretching programs

(continued)

G. R. Waryasz, MD, CSCS
Department of Orthopaedic Surgery, Massachusetts General Hospital, Boston, MA, USA

© Springer International Publishing AG, part of Springer Nature 2018   209
A. E. M. Eltorai et al. (eds.), *Essential Orthopedic Review*,
https://doi.org/10.1007/978-3-319-78387-1_94

(continued)

How much of the plantar fascia is released for chronic plantar fasciitis?	Medial 1/3–2/3. Do not perform a complete release
How is a plantar fascia rupture treated?	Cast or boot immobilization

Chapter 95
Morton Neuroma

Seth W. O'Donnell and Brad D. Blankenhorn

Which is the most common location for a Morton's Neuroma?	Between the third and fourth toes (third web space) of the foot
What structure frequently causes the compression?	Intermetatarsal ligament
What structures are frequently compressed?	Interdigital branches from both medial and lateral plantar nerves
What are the disadvantages to a plantar surgical approach?	Increased wound problems, painful scar on the weight bearing surface of the foot
What are some common nonoperative therapies?	Wide toe-box shoes, steroid injection, metatarsal pad

S. W. O'Donnell, MD (✉) · B. D. Blankenhorn, MD
Department of Orthopaedic Surgery, Warren Alpert Medical School of Brown University, Providence, RI, USA

© Springer International Publishing AG, part of Springer Nature 2018   211
A. E. M. Eltorai et al. (eds.), *Essential Orthopedic Review*,
https://doi.org/10.1007/978-3-319-78387-1_95

Chapter 96
Arthritic Foot

Seth W. O'Donnell and Brad D. Blankenhorn

What joints are fused in a triple fusion?	Subtalar, talo-navicular, calcaneo-cuboid
What is another term for the subtalar joint?	Talo-calcaneal joint
What is the difference between ankle arthrodesis and ankle arthroplasty?	Ankle arthrodesis involves a fusion of the tibio-talar joint; ankle arthroplasty involves replacing the tibio-talar joint with prosthetic implants
Which fractures can lead to increased risk of subtalar arthritis?	Calcaneal fractures
What is the major risk of joint fusion?	Abnormal loading of adjacent joints with degeneration

S. W. O'Donnell, MD (✉) · B. D. Blankenhorn, MD
Department of Orthopaedic Surgery, Warren Alpert Medical School of Brown University, Providence, RI, USA

© Springer International Publishing AG, part of Springer Nature 2018
A. E. M. Eltorai et al. (eds.), *Essential Orthopedic Review*,
https://doi.org/10.1007/978-3-319-78387-1_96

Chapter 97
Pelvic Ring Fractures

Daniel Brian Carlin Reid

What X-ray view is best for evaluating anterior/posterior translation of the hemipelvis, internal/external rotation of the hemipelvis, and SI joint widening?	Inlet view
What X-ray view is best for evaluating vertical translation of the hemipelvis and flexion-extension of the hemipelvis?	Outlet view
What is the most important ligamentous structure for pelvic stability?	Posterior sacroiliac ligamentous complex
What are the three main injury mechanism patterns described in the Young-Burgess classification?	Anterior posterior compression (APC), lateral compression (LC), vertical shear (VS)

(continued)

D. B. C. Reid, MD, MPH
Department of Orthopaedics, Rhode Island Hospital, Brown University, Providence, RI, USA

© Springer International Publishing AG, part of Springer Nature 2018   215
A. E. M. Eltorai et al. (eds.), *Essential Orthopedic Review*,
https://doi.org/10.1007/978-3-319-78387-1_97

(continued)

Injury to which structure differentiates between and APC-II and APC-III injury	Posterior sacroiliac ligamentous complex
What is the colloquial name for and LC-III injury?	Windswept pelvis (Ipsilateral LC injury with contralateral APC-type injury)
In general, which pelvic injury pattern is associated with the highest risk of bleeding and hypovolemic shock?	Vertical shear (VS)
What device can easily be applied in the emergency room to control pelvic hemorrhage in unstable pelvic ring injuries?	Pelvic binder
What anatomic landmark should a pelvic binder be centered over during application?	Greater trochanters
What fluoroscopic views best define the anterior-posterior and superior-inferior trajectories, respectively, for iliosacral screw placement?	Inlet view (anterior-posterior), outlet view, (superior-inferior)
What nerve root is at greatest risk when placing S1 iliosacral screws?	L5

Chapter 98
Acetabular Fractures

Daniel Brian Carlin Reid

What are the two oblique pelvis ("Judet") X-ray views and what do each view best?	Obturator oblique: Anterior column, posterior wall. Iliac oblique: Posterior column, anterior wall
What are the five "simple" types of acetabular fractures? (Letournal classification)	Posterior wall, posterior column, anterior wall, anterior column, transverse
What are the five "associated" types of acetabular fractures? (Letournal classification)	Posterior column/posterior wall, transverse/posterior wall, T-type, anterior column/posterior hemitransverse, associated both column
What feature defines an associated both column acetabular fracture?	Complete dissociation between acetabular articular surface and intact ilium

(continued)

D. B. C. Reid, MD, MPH
Department of Orthopaedics, Rhode Island Hospital,
Brown University, Providence, RI, USA

© Springer International Publishing AG, part of Springer Nature 2018   217
A. E. M. Eltorai et al. (eds.), *Essential Orthopedic Review*,
https://doi.org/10.1007/978-3-319-78387-1_98

(continued)

Name a common complication after operative fixation of acetabulum fractures and how it can be prevented.	Heterotopic ossification (HO). Prophylaxis can include radiation therapy or indomethacin
How can the lower extremity be positioned during surgery to minimize tension on the sciatic nerve?	Hip extension and knee flexion
What type of injury does the "spur sign" on the obturator oblique indicate and what does this sign represent?	Indicates associated both column acetabular fracture. Represents intact portion of iliac wing remaining in anatomic position as the acetabular dome and femoral head are translated medially

Part IV
Spine

Chapter 99
Vertebral Disc Disease

Dominic Kleinhenz

What is the function of the intervertebral disc?	Shock absorption and mobility
What are the components of the intervertebral disc?	Nucleus pulposus, anulus fibrosus
What types of collagen make up those components?	Type II (nucleus pulposus), Type I (anulus fibrosus)
How does water content in the disc change with aging?	It decreases
How does less water affect the disc?	It becomes weaker and more stiff

(continued)

D. Kleinhenz, MD
Rhode Island Hospital Orthopaedic Surgery Residency Program,
Warren Alpert School of Medicine of Brown University,
Providence, RI, USA

© Springer International Publishing AG, part of Springer Nature 2018   221
A. E. M. Eltorai et al. (eds.), *Essential Orthopedic Review*,
https://doi.org/10.1007/978-3-319-78387-1_99

(continued)

What is a disc protrusion?	Displaced nucleus that has not extended beyond the anulus
What is a disc extrusion?	Displaced nucleus through the anulus
What is a disc sequestration?	"Free fragment," displaced nucleus no longer in contact with disc
What nerve root(s) do central and paracentral disc herniations effect?	Traversing (L4/5 disc herniation leads to L5 radiculopathy)
What nerve root (s) do foraminal and extra-foraminal disc herniations effect?	Exiting (L4/5 disc herniation leads to L4 radiculopathy)

Chapter 100
Spondylolysis and Spondylolisthesis

Dominic Kleinhenz

What is the pars interarticularis?	Area between the superior and inferior intraarticular processes
What is spondylolysis?	A defect in the pars interarticularis
What X-ray views look for spondylolysis?	Right and left oblique
What are X-ray findings of spondylolysis?	"Scottie dog with a collar," lucency of the pars interarticularis seen on oblique views of the spine
What is the common clinical presentation for spondylosis?	A child or adolescent with back pain

(continued)

D. Kleinhenz, MD
Rhode Island Hospital Orthopaedic Surgery Residency Program,
Warren Alpert School of Medicine of Brown University,
Providence, RI, USA

© Springer International Publishing AG, part of Springer Nature 2018   223
A. E. M. Eltorai et al. (eds.), *Essential Orthopedic Review*,
https://doi.org/10.1007/978-3-319-78387-1_100

(continued)

What sport(s) have higher incidence of spondylosis?	Gymnastics and football. Sports with repetitive lumbar hyperextension
Most common exam finding in spondylolysis/ spondylolisthesis?	Hamstring tightness
What is spondylolisthesis?	Slippage of one vertebral body on another
What are the types of spondylolisthesis?	Isthmic, degenerative, traumatic
What type of spondylolisthesis is caused by the defect in the pars?	Isthmic

Chapter 101
Spinal Stenosis

Dominic Kleinhenz

What is spinal stenosis?	Narrowing of the spinal canal leading to pressure on the neural elements
What defines cervical stenosis?	Absolute cervical stenosis is defined by canal diameter <10 mm. Relative cervical stenosis is defined by canal diameter between 10 and 13 mm
What structures are pathologic in lumbar spinal stenosis?	Intervertebral disc, ligamentum flavum, facet joints
What is neurogenic claudication?	A common symptom of spinal stenosis. Onset of bilateral buttock or leg pain after walking a certain distance

(continued)

D. Kleinhenz, MD
Rhode Island Hospital Orthopaedic Surgery Residency Program,
Warren Alpert School of Medicine of Brown University,
Providence, RI, USA

© Springer International Publishing AG, part of Springer Nature 2018   225
A. E. M. Eltorai et al. (eds.), *Essential Orthopedic Review*,
https://doi.org/10.1007/978-3-319-78387-1_101

(continued)

How do you differentiate neurogenic and vascular claudication?	Examining peripheral pulses
What is the "shopping cart" sign?	Patients with spinal stenosis typically feel better in a flexed position. Thus, they feel better when leaning forward on the shopping cart
Why do patients with spinal stenosis feel better in flexion?	Flexion tightens the hypertrophied ligamentum flavum taking some pressure off the thecal sac
Which nerve root is most commonly affected in spinal stenosis?	L5
Where can the L5 nerve root be compressed?	Centrally or in the lateral recess at L4/5, or in the L5/S1 foramen or extra-foraminal zone

Chapter 102
Spinal Cord Injury

Jacob Babu

What should be done on the field for a football player with concern of cervical spine injury?	Spinal precautions/stabilization, leave helmet in place, remove facemask
What tract is responsible for relaying pain and temperature sensation from the body to the brain?	Spinothalamic tract

(continued)

J. Babu, MD, MHA
Department of Orthopaedic Surgery, Warren Alpert Medical School of Brown University, Rhode Island Hospital, Providence, RI, USA
e-mail: jacob_babu@brown.edu

© Springer International Publishing AG, part of Springer Nature 2018 227
A. E. M. Eltorai et al. (eds.), *Essential Orthopedic Review*,
https://doi.org/10.1007/978-3-319-78387-1_102

(continued)

What American Spinal Injury Association (ASIA) grade is a SCI injury that leaves a patient with no motor function, but preserved anal sensation?	A: Complete injury: No preserved sensory or motor function, including in sacral segments B: Sensory incomplete: Complete motor deficits distal to the neurological level, but some sensory is preserved. Sensation is preserved in the anal region and patient may recognize light touch or pin prick in this area C: Motor incomplete: Motor preservation with less than half of the key muscles below the level of injury having a muscle grade of 3 or above. Voluntary anal contraction is found on physical exam D: Motor incomplete: Motor preservation with half or more of the key muscles below the level of injury having a muscle grade of 3 or above E: Normal sensation and motor throughout
What level of spinal cord injury results in need for mechanical ventilation?	Injury to C3 or above
What physical exam maneuver can help identify if a patient is in spinal shock?	Loss of the bulbocavernosus reflex
Decreased blood pressure and decreased heart rate is consistent with what type of shock?	Neurogenic shock

What should the mean arterial pressure (MAP) be maintained at or above to prevent further ischemic damage to the spinal cord?	MAPs >85 mmHg
What preexisting condition predisposes a patient to central cord syndrome?	Cervical central stenosis/spondylosis
Which spinal cord injury pattern results in preservation of the dorsal columns, with loss of motor and sensory function below the level of injury?	Anterior cord injury
Which incomplete spinal cord injury pattern is associated with the greatest prognosis for functional recovery?	Brown-Sequard syndrome

Chapter 103
Cervical Fracture/Dislocation

Jacob Babu

Why is spinal cord injury more common in fracture/dislocations of the subaxial (C3-C7) cervical spine than at C1/C2?	The spinal canal is much larger proximally
What are some radiographic parameters that help identify occipitocervical dissociation?	The power ratio, basion-dens interval, basion-axial interval
What ligament is the key component to maintaining stability in C1 atlas fractures?	The transverse atlantal ligament (TAL)
What type of odontoid fracture is most likely to go on to a nonunion?	Type 2 fracture

(continued)

J. Babu, MD, MHA
Department of Orthopaedic Surgery, Warren Alpert Medical School of Brown University, Rhode Island Hospital, Providence, RI, USA
e-mail: jacob_babu@brown.edu

© Springer International Publishing AG, part of Springer Nature 2018   231
A. E. M. Eltorai et al. (eds.), *Essential Orthopedic Review*,
https://doi.org/10.1007/978-3-319-78387-1_103

(continued)

What conditions should increase the practitioners level of concern for radiographically occult or minimally displaced cervical spine fractures?	Ankylosing spondylitis, diffuse idiopathic skeletal hyperostosis (DISH), ossification of the posterior longitudinal ligament
What axial CT scan finding is suggestive of jumped cervical facets?	Reverse hamburger sign—articular surface of facets are no longer in contact
What should be done for an identified cervical facet dislocation and progressive neurological worsening in the alert and cooperative patient?	Emergent closed reduction with sequential traction

Chapter 104
Thoracolumbar Fracture

Jacob Babu

What is the normal range of thoracic kyphosis?	20–50°
At what level does the spinal cord terminate and continue as the cauda equina?	L1-L2
The integrity of what structure suggests possibly maintained stability in the thoracolumbar spine despite sustaining a burst fracture?	The posterior ligamentous complex
What other injury occurs with high frequency concomitantly with flexion-distraction injuries or "seat belt injuries"?	Abdominal viscera injuries

(continued)

J. Babu, MD, MHA
Department of Orthopaedic Surgery, Warren Alpert Medical
School of Brown University, Rhode Island Hospital,
Providence, RI, USA
e-mail: jacob_babu@brown.edu

© Springer International Publishing AG, part of Springer Nature 2018   233
A. E. M. Eltorai et al. (eds.), *Essential Orthopedic Review*,
https://doi.org/10.1007/978-3-319-78387-1_104

(continued)

What scoring system helps guide practitioners on whether to manage thoracolumbar fractures operatively vs. nonoperatively?	The Thoracolumbar Injury Classification and Severity Score (TLICS)
What deformity does a practitioner monitor for with radiographs at follow up when managing a patient with a 2–3 column fracture nonoperatively?	Progressive kyphosis
What is the potential etiology of progressive neurologic deficits in a spine fracture suffered by a patient with ankylosis spondylitis or DISH?	Epidural hematoma—especially when anticoagulated
What is the greatest predictor of a patient suffering a vertebral compression fracture in the future?	Prior vertebral compression fractures
What medical management can help prevent future vertebral compression, fragility fractures?	Bisphosphonates

Chapter 105
Lumbar Spine Conditions

Eren O. Kuris

What percentage of the general population will experience low back pain at some point in their lifetime?	54–80%
What is the most common cause of low back pain?	Muscle strain
What percentage of low back pain resolves within 1 year?	90%
What are risk factors for low back pain?	Obesity

(continued)

E. O. Kuris, MD
Department of Orthopaedic Surgery, Warren Alpert Medical School of Brown University, Providence, RI, USA

© Springer International Publishing AG, part of Springer Nature 2018   235
A. E. M. Eltorai et al. (eds.), *Essential Orthopedic Review*,
https://doi.org/10.1007/978-3-319-78387-1_105

(continued)

What is the differential diagnosis for low back pain?	Muscle strain Disk herniation Spinal stenosis Lumbar radiculopathy Abdominal aortic aneurysm Degenerative spinal conditions (such as spondylolisthesis)
When should you order imaging for low back pain?	If pain persists and does not respond to conservative treatment options (such as activity modification, NSAIDs, physical therapy)
What are some red flags that indicate that imaging should be obtained sooner?	Signs or symptoms of infection (fever, chills, etc) History of cancer Trauma Neurologic symptoms Symptoms concerning for cauda equina syndrome (bowel or bladder changes)
What are Waddell signs?	A system used to evaluate a patient for non-organic causes of back pain – superficial and non-anatomic tenderness – excessive verbalization or gesturing of pain – nonanatomic motor or sensory impairment – pain with axial compression or simulated rotation of spine – negative straight leg raise when patient is distracted

The presence of three or more of these findings suggests a non-organic cause of the patient's low back pain

Suggested Reading

1. Biyani A, Andersson GB. Low back pain: pathophysiology and management. J Am Acad Orthop Surg. 2004;12(2):106–15. Review. PubMed PMID: 15089084.
2. Herkowitz HN, Garfin SR, Eismont FJ, Bel GR, Balderston RA. Rothman-Simeone The spine. 6th ed. Philadelphia, PA: Saunders; 2011.
3. Shen FH, Samartzis D, Andersson GB. Nonsurgical management of acute and chronic low back pain. J Am Acad Orthop Surg. 2006;14(8):477–87. Review. PubMed PMID: 16885479.
4. Waddell G, McCulloch JA, Kummel E, Venner RM. Nonorganic physical signs in low-back pain. Spine (Phila Pa 1976). 1980;5(2):117–25. PubMed PMID:6446157.

Chapter 106
Adult Spinal Deformity

Dominic Kleinhenz

What are the normal sagittal curves of the spine?	Lumbar lordosis, thoracic kyphosis, cervical lordosis
What is sagittal vertical axis?	Measurement of sagittal balance; plumb line from center of C7 to vertical line from posterosuperior corner of S1
What measurement defines abnormal positive sagittal balance?	Greater than 5 cm sagittal vertical axis, PT > 20°, PI-LL > 10°
What is pelvic incidence?	Angle formed between a line drawn from the center of the femoral heads and a line perpendicular to the sacral endplate drawn from its midpoint

(continued)

D. Kleinhenz, MD
Rhode Island Hospital Orthopaedic Surgery Residency Program, Warren Alpert School of Medicine of Brown University, Providence, RI, USA

© Springer International Publishing AG, part of Springer Nature 2018   239
A. E. M. Eltorai et al. (eds.), *Essential Orthopedic Review*,
https://doi.org/10.1007/978-3-319-78387-1_106

(continued)

Why is pelvic incidence important?	It is a fixed pelvic parameter; it varies from person to person, but does not change with positioning of spine or pelvis
How is lumbar lordosis measured?	A cobb angle is drawn from superior endplate of L1 and caudal endplate of L5
What is the relationship between pelvic incidence and lumbar lordosis?	Pelvic incidence should match lumbar lordosis within 10°
How do patients compensate for abnormal sagittal balance?	Through retroversion of their pelvis and hip and knee flexion
Why are patients with adult spinal deformity worse at end of day?	Patients lose their ability to compensate throughout the day

Chapter 107
Spine Tumors

Eren O. Kuris

What is the most common tumor of the spine?	Metastatic disease
What primary tumors most frequently metastasize to bone?	Breast, prostate, lung, kidney, and thyroid
What percentage of spinal column tumors are from metastatic disease?	97%
Where is the most common site of bony metastasis from a malignancy?	Spine, specifically, the thoracic spine (second most common is proximal femur)
What other conditions are associated with spine tumors?	Multiple myeloma Lymphoma

(continued)

E. O. Kuris, MD
Department of Orthopaedic Surgery, Warren Alpert Medical School of Brown University, Providence, RI, USA

© Springer International Publishing AG, part of Springer Nature 2018   241
A. E. M. Eltorai et al. (eds.), *Essential Orthopedic Review*,
https://doi.org/10.1007/978-3-319-78387-1_107

(continued)

What scoring system can determine life expectancy in a patient with spine metastasis?	Takuhashi scoring system
When is palliative treatment recommended?	
When the life expectancy is less than 6 months	
What are the goals of treatment for metastatic spine lesions?	Neurological decompression Surgical stabilization
What adjuvant treatment can be used either before or after surgery?	Radiation
If a patient has metastatic renal cell carcinoma, what procedure should the patient undergo before surgical resection and stabilization of the lesion?	Preoperative embolization to minimize bleeding
Where do most malignant tumors occur in the spine vertebrae	Anteriorly (vertebral body)
Where do most benign spine tumors occur?	Posterior elements
What are some primary benign spine tumors?	Osteoblastoma/Osteoid Osteoma Giant cell tumor Aneurysmal bone cyst Osteochondroma Hemangioma
What are some primary malignant spine tumors?	Chordoma Osteosarcoma Ewing's sarcoma Chondrosarcoma

How do you distinguish between osteoid osteoma and osteoblastoma?	Size (<2 cm in diameter is osteoid osteoma; >2 cm is osteoblastoma)
How is an osteoid osteoma/osteoblastoma commonly found in children?	Painful scoliosis (nonrotational)
Where do osteoid osteoma and osteoblastoma usually occur in the spine?	Posterior vertebral elements
What is the most common primary malignant spine tumor in adults?	Chordoma
What is the most common site for a chordoma?	Sacrum and coccyx (50% of chordomas)
What are the histological features?	Vacuolated physaliferous cells with a foamy appearance
What is the 5-year survival rate in patients with chordoma?	60%

Suggested Reading

1. Herkowitz HN, Garfin SR, Eismont FJ, Bel GR, Balderston RA. Rothman-Simeone The spine. 6th ed. Philadelphia, PA: Saunders; 2011.
2. Schwab JH, Healey JH, Rose P, et al. The surgical management of sacral chordomas. Spine. 2009;34:2700–4.
3. Tokuhashi Y, Ajiro Y, Umezawa N. Outcome of treatment for spinal metastases using scoring system for preoperative evaluation of prognosis. Spine (Phila Pa 1976). 2009;34(1):69–73. https://doi.org/10.1097/BRS.0b013e3181913f19. PubMed PMID: 19127163.

Chapter 108
Spine Infections

Eren O. Kuris

What are the various types of spine infections?	Spinal epidural abscess
	Vertebral osteomyelitis
	Discitis
	Granulomatous infections (such as spinal tuberculosis)
	Postoperative wound infections
	Spinal Intradural infections

(continued)

E. O. Kuris, MD
Department of Orthopaedic Surgery, Warren Alpert Medical
School of Brown University, Providence, RI, USA

© Springer International Publishing AG, part of Springer Nature 2018   245
A. E. M. Eltorai et al. (eds.), *Essential Orthopedic Review*,
https://doi.org/10.1007/978-3-319-78387-1_108

(continued)

What are risk factors for spine infections?	History of IV drug use
	Immunocompromised state
	Malignancy
	Diabetes
	Malnutrition
	Recent systemic infection
	History of spinal procedure
	History of travel to an endemic region
	Immunosuppressive medications
What is the most common pathogen?	*Staphylococcus aureus*
What pathogen may be present in patients with a history of IV drug use?	*Pseudomonas aeruginosa*
What is a spinal epidural abscess?	A bacterial infection of the spine that leads to a collection of pus between the dura and the tissue around it
How can spine infections present?	Systemic symptoms (such as fevers, chills, malaise)
	Pain (can be acute or insidious onset)
	Physical examination may reveal neurological deficits in severe cases (such as radiculopathy, myelopathy, or cauda equina syndrome)

What labs should be ordered in the work-up of spine infections?	– WBC count – ESR – CRP – If there is concern for a systemic infection, consider chest X-ray, blood cultures, and a urinalysis
What imaging study is generally the gold standard for the evaluation of spine infections?	MRI with gadolinium contrast
When should you begin antibiotics?	After cultures have been obtained, unless the patient is systemically ill or has risk of neurological deterioration
What is the treatment for spinal epidural abscess?	Surgical decompression with or without stabilization
What is the first line of treatment for vertebral osteomyelitis?	Bracing with an extended course of IV antibiotics (after a pathogen has been identified through blood cultures or biopsy)
How can you monitor the activity of spine infections?	Serial inflammatory markers, such as ESR and CRP

Suggested Reading

1. Darouiche RO. Spinal epidural abscess. N Engl J Med. 2006;355(19):2012–20. Review. PubMed PMID: 17093252.
2. Herkowitz HN, Garfin SR, Eismont FJ, Bel GR, Balderston RA. Rothman-Simeone The spine. 6th ed. Philadelphia, PA: Saunders; 2011.
3. Tay BK, Deckey J, Hu SS. Spinal infections. J Am Acad Orthop Surg. 2002;10(3):188–97. Review. PubMed PMID: 12041940.

Part V
Pediatric Orthopedics

Chapter 109
Angular Variations

Heather Hansen

What exam components are including in the rotational profile?	Foot-progression angle, internal and external rotation of the hips, thigh-foot angle, and any foot deformities
What is the foot-progression angle?	A measurement of the degree of intoeing or outtoeing compared to an imaginary straight line on the floor
What does the internal and external rotation of the hip measure?	The femoral rotational variation/torsion
What is the thigh-foot angle and what does it measure?	With the child prone, the angle between the axis of the thigh and the axis of the foot with the foot held in a neutral position. It measures tibial torsion

(continued)

H. Hansen, MD
Division of Pediatric Orthopaedic Surgery, Department of Orthopaedics, The Warren Alpert Medical School of Brown University, Providence, RI, USA
e-mail: hdh418@mail.usask.ca

© Springer International Publishing AG, part of Springer Nature 2018   251
A. E. M. Eltorai et al. (eds.), *Essential Orthopedic Review*,
https://doi.org/10.1007/978-3-319-78387-1_109

(continued)

What is the typical progression of the tibiofemoral angle in a young child?	Genu varum (bowlegged) as infant, genu valgum (knock-kneed) from age 2 to 4
What is the average adult tibiofemoral angle?	7° of valgus
What are some benign causes of intoeing?	Metatarsus adductus, increased or persistent internal tibial torsion, or increased or persistent femoral anteversion
What are some pathologic causes of intoeing?	Cerebral palsy, infantile Blount's, metabolic bone disease, skeletal dysplasias
What are the main surgical strategies for symptomatic angular variations?	Guided growth or osteotomies

Bibliography

1. Aronsson DD, Lisle JW. The pediatric orthopaedic examination. In: Weinstein SL, editor. Lovell and Winter's pediatric orthopaedics, vol. 1. 7th ed. Philadelphia: Wolters Kluwer; 2014. p. 91–5. Print.
2. Birch JG. The orthopaedic examination: a comprehensive overview. In: Herring JA, editor. Tachjian's pediatric orthopaedics: from the Texas Scottish Rite Hospital, vol. 1. 5th ed. Philadelphia: Elsevier Saunders; 2014a. p. 25–6. Print.
3. Birch JG. The orthopaedic examination: clinical application. In: Herring JA, editor. Tachjian's pediatric orthopaedics: from the Texas Scottish Rite Hospital, vol. 1. 5th ed. Philadelphia: Elsevier Saunders; 2014b. p. 63–4. Print.
4. Lincoln TL, Suen PW. Common rotational variations in children. J Am Acad Orthop Surg. 2003;11:312–20.

Chapter 110
Pediatric Fractures: Management Principles

Aristides I. Cruz Jr

What are the minimum number of views one should order when evaluating a fractured extremity?	Two (typically AP and lateral)
What is the most common fracture reported in children?	Distal radius
Which specific types of fractures are associated with abuse/non-accidental trauma?	Metaphyseal corner fractures, long bone fractures in child of non-walking age, posterior rib fractures, distal humerus transphyseal fracture, multiple fractures in various stages of healing

(continued)

A. I. Cruz Jr., MD, MBA
Department of Orthopaedic Surgery, Warren Alpert Medical School of Brown University, Providence, RI, USA

© Springer International Publishing AG, part of Springer Nature 2018   253
A. E. M. Eltorai et al. (eds.), *Essential Orthopedic Review*,
https://doi.org/10.1007/978-3-319-78387-1_110

(continued)

Through which physeal zone do Salter-Harris I fractures typically occur?	Zone of hypertrophy
Which clinical finding is most indicative of impending compartment syndrome in a child?	Increasing pain medicine requirement
What are Harris growth arrest lines?	These lines result from a temporary slowdown of normal longitudinal growth after injury or illness and appear as transversely oriented, sclerotic lines on plain X-ray and usually duplicate the contiguous physeal contour

Chapter 111
Radial Head Dislocation

Aristides I. Cruz Jr.

What is a Monteggia fracture?	Ulnar shaft fracture associated with radial head dislocation
What is the Bado classification scheme?	Describes Monteggia fractures relative to direction of radial head dislocation. Type I: Anterior dislocation Type II: Posterior dislocation Type III: Lateral dislocation Type IV: Dislocation + radius fracture
What is the treatment for asymptomatic congenital radial head dislocation?	Observation

(continued)

A. I. Cruz Jr., MD, MBA
Department of Orthopaedic Surgery, Warren Alpert Medical School of Brown University, Providence, RI, USA

© Springer International Publishing AG, part of Springer Nature 2018   255
A. E. M. Eltorai et al. (eds.), *Essential Orthopedic Review*,
https://doi.org/10.1007/978-3-319-78387-1_111

(continued)

Which direction is the radial head most commonly dislocated in congenital radial head dislocation?	Posterior
Which motion(s) is/are most commonly lost in congenital radial head dislocation?	Elbow extension/forearm supination
Which radiographic line should be measured when evaluating for radial head dislocation?	Radiocapitellar line

Chapter 112
Slipped Capital Femoral Epiphysis

Heather Hansen

What are risk factors for SCFE?	Obesity, polynesian ancestry, endocrinopathies, radiation therapy, renal osteodystrophy, Down syndrome
What is the more useful classification of SCFE?	Stable vs. unstable, acute vs. chronic
What defines an unstable SCFE?	Inability to weight bear, even with crutches
What is a major concern with unstable SCFEs?	Osteonecrosis of the femoral head
What are the common findings of SCFE?	Hip/groin pain, limp, decreased range of motion of the hip, and KNEE or THIGH pain

(continued)

H. Hansen, MD
Division of Pediatric Orthopaedic Surgery, Department of
Orthopaedics, Alpert Medical School of Brown University,
Providence, RI, USA

© Springer International Publishing AG, part of Springer Nature 2018   257
A. E. M. Eltorai et al. (eds.), *Essential Orthopedic Review*,
https://doi.org/10.1007/978-3-319-78387-1_112

(continued)

What is the obligate external rotation sign?	The hip automatically falls into external rotation with hip flexion
What radiographic view is most sensitive for detecting SCFEs?	Lateral view
What is Klein's line?	A line drawn tangential to the superior femoral neck on the lateral hip radiograph
What is the presumed natural history of a severe slip?	Development of osteoarthritis
What is the current accepted treatment of SCFEs?	Operative fixation

Bibliography

1. Kay RM, Kim Y-J. Slipped capital femoral epiphysis. In: Weinstein SL, editor. Lovell and Winter's pediatric orthopaedics, vol. 2. 7th ed. Philadelphia: Wolters Kluwer; 2014. p. 1165–221. Print.
2. Herring JA. Slipped capital femoral epiphysis. In: Herring JA, editor. Tachjian's pediatric orthopaedics: from the Texas Scottish Rite Hospital, vol. 2. 5th ed. Philadelphia: Elsevier Saunders; 2014. p. 630–65. Print.
3. Thawrani DP, Feldman DS, Sala DA. Current practice in the management of slipped capital femoral epiphysis. J Pediatr Orthop. 2016;36(3):e27–37.
4. Aronsson DD, Loder RT, Breur GJ. Slipped capital femoral epiphysis: current concepts. J Am Acad Orthop Surg. 2006;14(12):666–79.

Chapter 113
Congenital Hip Dislocation

Jose M. Ramirez

What are risk factors for CHD?	First born, breech, family history, female, oligohydramnios
What is the Barlow exam maneuver?	Dislocation of flexed, adducted femur with axial load
What is the ortolani exam maneuver?	Reduction of dislocated hip with flexion, elevation, and abduction
What is a normal alpha angle?	Greater than 60°
What is the preferred treatment of a reducible hip in a patient <6 months of age?	Pavlik harness

J. M. Ramirez, MD
Department of Orthopaedic Surgery, Alpert Medical School of Brown University, Providence, RI, USA

© Springer International Publishing AG, part of Springer Nature 2018   259
A. E. M. Eltorai et al. (eds.), *Essential Orthopedic Review*,
https://doi.org/10.1007/978-3-319-78387-1_113

Chapter 114
Congenital Coxa Vara

Jose M. Ramirez

What is a normal femoral neck shaft angle?	125–135°
What is Hilgenreiner's angle?	Angle formed between Hilgenreiner's line and proximal femoral physis
What surgery is typically indicated for Hilgenreiner epiphyseal angle >60°?	Corrective valgus derotational osteotomy

J. M. Ramirez, MD
Department of Orthopaedic Surgery, Alpert Medical School
of Brown University, Providence, RI, USA

© Springer International Publishing AG, part of Springer Nature 2018   261
A. E. M. Eltorai et al. (eds.), *Essential Orthopedic Review*,
https://doi.org/10.1007/978-3-319-78387-1_114

Chapter 115
Osteochondrosis (Osgood-Schlatter and Osteochondritis Dissecans)

Jose M. Ramirez

What is the most common location for OCD in the upper extremity of a young athlete?	Capitellum
What is the most common location for OCD of the knee?	Medial femoral condyle
What is Sinding-Larsen Johansson syndrome?	Chronic apophysitis of inferior pole of the patella
What can be seen on radiographs of the knee in Osgood-Schlatter's disease?	Fragmentation of the tibial tubercle
What is Iselin's disease?	Apophysitis of base of fifth metatarsal

J. M. Ramirez, MD
Department of Orthopaedic Surgery, Alpert Medical School
of Brown University, Providence, RI, USA

© Springer International Publishing AG, part of Springer Nature 2018   263
A. E. M. Eltorai et al. (eds.), *Essential Orthopedic Review*,
https://doi.org/10.1007/978-3-319-78387-1_115

Chapter 116
Osteogenesis Imperfecta (OI)

Jose M. Ramirez

OI is caused by a qualitative and/or quantitative defect in what protein?	Type 1 Collagen
What medical therapy can reduce fracture rate in OI?	Bisphosphonate therapy
Signs of myelopathy on exam should raise concern for what complication associated with OI?	Basilar invagination
What upper extremity fracture is pathognomonic for OI?	Olecranon apophyseal avulsion fracture
What lower extremity deformity associated with OI can lead to a Trendelenburg gait?	Coxa Vara

J. M. Ramirez, MD
Department of Orthopaedic Surgery, Alpert Medical School of Brown University, Providence, RI, USA

© Springer International Publishing AG, part of Springer Nature 2018   265
A. E. M. Eltorai et al. (eds.), *Essential Orthopedic Review*,
https://doi.org/10.1007/978-3-319-78387-1_116

Chapter 117
Child Abuse

Jose M. Ramirez

What is the chance of death for a child who is a victim of unreported physical abuse?	5–10%
What is the classically reported location for concerning extremity fractures in child abuse?	Metaphyseal corner fractures
What elbow injury should raise concern for child abuse?	Distal humerus physeal separation
What is the most common presenting sign in an abused child?	Skin lesion
True/False: Physicians are legally obligated to report cases of child abuse.	True

J. M. Ramirez, MD
Department of Orthopaedic Surgery, Alpert Medical School
of Brown University, Providence, RI, USA

© Springer International Publishing AG, part of Springer Nature 2018   267
A. E. M. Eltorai et al. (eds.), *Essential Orthopedic Review*,
https://doi.org/10.1007/978-3-319-78387-1_117

Chapter 118
Legg-Calve-Perthes Disease

Jose M. Ramirez

What are the Waldenström stages of Perthes disease?	Initial, fragmentation, reossification, remodeling (healing)
What is the crescent sign?	Radiographically, a subchondral fracture of femoral head
What syndrome should be in the differential diagnosis of a patient suspected bilateral perthes disease?	Multiple epiphyseal dysplasia (MED)
When does fragmentation typically occur?	Approximately 6 months after the onset of symptoms

J. M. Ramirez, MD
Department of Orthopaedic Surgery, Alpert Medical School
of Brown University, Providence, RI, USA

© Springer International Publishing AG, part of Springer Nature 2018   269
A. E. M. Eltorai et al. (eds.), *Essential Orthopedic Review*,
https://doi.org/10.1007/978-3-319-78387-1_118

Chapter 119
Cerebral Palsy

Heather Hansen

What is the term used to describe the brain lesion in cerebral palsy?	Static encephalopathy
When does the brain insult occur?	Prenatally, perinatally, or during childhood
What is the time course of musculoskeletal pathology?	Progressive
What is the name of the most common measurement of gross motor function?	Gross Motor Function Classification System (GMFCS)

(continued)

H. Hansen, MD
Division of Pediatric Orthopaedic Surgery,
Department of Orthopaedics,
Alpert Medical School of Brown University,
Providence, RI, USA

© Springer International Publishing AG, part of Springer Nature 2018   271
A. E. M. Eltorai et al. (eds.), *Essential Orthopedic Review*,
https://doi.org/10.1007/978-3-319-78387-1_119

(continued)

What are some risk factors for the development of CP?	Low birth weight/prematurity, maternal infection, drug/alcohol abuse, congenital brain malformation, perinatal anoxia, breech presentation, post-natal infections, or head trauma
What is the main treatment option for a fixed musculotendinous contracture?	Tendon lengthening
What is responsible for hip subluxation?	Muscle imbalance between spasticity and contracture of the adductors and flexors that overpower the weaker and noncontracted hip extensors and abductors
What are the three surgical categories of treatment of a hip at risk of subluxation/dislocation?	(1) soft tissue release for subluxation or a hip at risk, (2) reduction and reconstruction of the subluxated or dislocated hip, and (3) salvage surgery for long-standing painful dislocations
What is the most common spine problem in cerebral palsy?	Scoliosis
What is the typical appearance of a scoliosis curve?	Long, sweeping, C-shaped

Bibliography

1. Kerr Graham H, Thomason P, Novacheck TF. Cerebral palsy. In: Weinstein SL, editor. Lovell and Winter's pediatric orthopaedics, vol. 1. 7th ed. Philadelphia: Wolters Kluwer; 2014. p. 486–554. Print.

2. Karol LA. Disorders of the brain. In: Herring JA, editor. Tachjian's pediatric orthopaedics: from the Texas Scottish Rite Hospital, vol. 2. 5th ed. Philadelphia: Elsevier Saunders; 2014. p. 370–85. Print.
3. Refakis CA, Baldwin KD, Speigel DA, Sankar WN. Treatment of the dislocated hip in infants with spasticity. J Pediatr Orthop. 2016 [Epub ahead of print].
4. Aversano MW, Sheikh Taha AM, Mundluru S, Otsuka NY. What's new in the orthopedic treatment of cerebral palsy. J Pediatr Orthop. 2017;31(3):210–6.
5. McCarthy JJ, D'Andrea LP, Betz RR. Scoliosis in the child with cerebral palsy. J Am Acad Orthop Surg. 2006;14(6):367–75.
6. Karol LA. Surgical management of the lower extremity in ambulatory children with cerebral palsy. J Am Acad Orthop Surg. 2004;12(3):196–203.

Chapter 120
Spinal Bifida

Daniel Brian Carlin Reid

Supplementation of what vitamin can decrease risk of spina bifida?	Folate
What lab test can be obtained in the second trimester to evaluate for spina bifida	Alpha-fetoprotein (usually elevated in spina bifida)
What is the most common comorbid condition with spina bifida?	Type II Arnold-Chiari Malformation
What allergy is common in patients with spina bifida?	Latex
Why is L4 considered a "key level" for function in patients with spina bifida?	Important for quadriceps function, allows some independent community ambulation

(continued)

D. B. C. Reid, MD, MPH
Department of Orthopaedics,
Rhode Island Hospital, Brown University,
Providence, RI, USA

© Springer International Publishing AG, part of Springer Nature 2018   275
A. E. M. Eltorai et al. (eds.), *Essential Orthopedic Review*,
https://doi.org/10.1007/978-3-319-78387-1_120

(continued)

Rapid scoliosis curve progression in patient's with spina bifida should raise concern for what?	Tethered cord and/or hydrocephalus
What should be ordered in patients with spina bifida presenting with warm, red, swollen joints (other than infectious workup)?	X-rays (pathologic fractures common in myelodysplastic children, often mistaken for infection)

Chapter 121
Charcot-Marie-Tooth Disease

Heather Hansen and Seth W. O'Donnell

What is Charcot-Marie-Tooth (CMT) disease?	Hereditary motor-sensory neuropathy
What is the common foot deformity seen with progressive CMT?	Cavo-varus
What muscle imbalances result from CMT?	Weak tibialis anterior is overpowered by peroneus longus; weak peroneus brevis is overpowered by tibialis posterior
Other than the foot and ankle, what orthopedic manifestations of CMT may be present?	Hip dysplasia, scoliosis, wasting of the hand intrinsic muscles

(continued)

H. Hansen, MD (✉) · S. W. O'Donnell, MD
Division of Pediatric Orthopaedic Surgery,
Department of Orthopaedics,
Alpert Medical School of Brown University,
Providence, RI, USA

© Springer International Publishing AG, part of Springer Nature 2018 277
A. E. M. Eltorai et al. (eds.), *Essential Orthopedic Review*,
https://doi.org/10.1007/978-3-319-78387-1_121

(continued)

What is often the first foot abnormality seen in CMT?	Plantar flexion of the first ray
What test can be used to assess the rigidity of a hindfoot deformity?	Coleman block test
What is a cavus foot?	A pathologically high arch
What does "equinus" describe?	The amount of plantar flexion at the ankle; often due to a contracture of the Achilles tendon or gastroc-soleus complex
What are diagnostic tests to perform to confirm diagnosis?	Nerve conduction studies, electromyography (EMG), and genetic testing. Nerve biopsy provides definitive diagnosis but often isn't necessary

Bibliography

1. Thompson GH, Berenson FR. Other neuromuscular disorders. In: Weinstein SL, editor. Lovell and Winter's pediatric orthopaedics, vol. 2. 7th ed. Philadelphia: Wolters Kluwer; 2014. p. 610–5. Print.
2. Podeszwa DA. Disorders of the peripheral nervous system. In: Herring JA, editor. Tachjian's pediatric orthopaedics: from the Texas Scottish Rite Hospital, vol. 2. 5th ed. Philadelphia: Elsevier Saunders; 2014. p. 285–97. Print.
3. Casare F, Francesco T, Matteo N, Antonio M, Carlotta C, Daniele F, Camilla P, Sandro G. Surgical treatment of cavus foot in Charcot-Marie-Tooth disease: a review of twenty-four cases: AAOS exhibit selection. J Bone Joint Surg Am. 2015;97(6):e30.

4. Schwend Richard M, Drennan JC. Cavus foot deformity in children. J Am Acad Orthop Surg. 2003;11:201–11.
5. Nagai MK, Chan G, Guille JT, Kumar SJ, Scavina M, Mackenzie WG. Prevalence of Charcot-Marie-Tooth disease in patients who have bilateral cavovarus feet. J Pediatr Orthop. 2006;26(4):438–43.
6. Yagerman SE, Cross MB, Green DW, Scher DM. Pediatric orthopedic conditions in Charcot-Marie-Tooth disease: a literature review. Curr Opin Pediatr. 2012;24(1):50–60.

Chapter 122
Muscular Dystrophy

Jose M. Ramirez

What protein is defective in MD?	Dystrophin
What is the inheritance pattern of MD?	X-linked recessive
How does Becker's MD differ from Duchenne's MD?	Becker's is related to a decrease in dystrophin
What is Gower's sign?	Rising by using arms to compensate for weakness or core muscles
What foot abnormality is seen in MD?	Equinovarus foot

J. M. Ramirez, MD
Department of Orthopaedic Surgery, Alpert Medical School
of Brown University, Providence, RI, USA

© Springer International Publishing AG, part of Springer Nature 2018   281
A. E. M. Eltorai et al. (eds.), *Essential Orthopedic Review*,
https://doi.org/10.1007/978-3-319-78387-1_122

Chapter 123
Arthrogryposis

Jonathan R. Schiller

What is the common position of the upper extremities?	Shoulder abdducted internally rotated; elbow extended; wrist flexed with ulnar deviation
What is the common position of the lower extremities?	Hips flexed abducted and externally rotated; knees typically extended; clubfeet
What type of clubfoot deformity is present in arthrogryposis?	Rigid, requiring surgical release

(continued)

J. R. Schiller, MD
Adolescent and Young Adult Hip Program, Orthopaedic Surgery,
The Warren Alpert School of Medicine of Brown University,
Providence, RI, USA

Division of Pediatric Orthopaedics and Scoliosis,
Hasbro Children's Hospital, Rhode Island Hospital,
Providence, RI, USA

Division of Sports Medicine,
Hasbro Children's Hospital, Rhode Island Hospital,
Providence, RI, USA
e-mail: jonathan_schiller@brown.edu

© Springer International Publishing AG, part of Springer Nature 2018   283
A. E. M. Eltorai et al. (eds.), *Essential Orthopedic Review*,
https://doi.org/10.1007/978-3-319-78387-1_123

(continued)

| What is the most common type of spine deformity? | C-shaped neuromuscular pattern |
| What is the inheritance pattern of arthrogryposis multiplex congenita? | Autosomal recessive |

Chapter 124
Achondroplasia

Heather Hansen

What is the most common form of dwarfism?	Achondroplasia
What zone of the growth plate is affected?	Provisional calcification
What gene is involved?	Fibroblast growth factor 3 (FGFR3)
What is the inheritance pattern?	Autosomal dominant
What appearance do achondroplastic hands have?	Trident
What appearance do the knees typically have?	Genu varum

(continued)

H. Hansen, MD
Division of Pediatric Orthopaedic Surgery,
Department of Orthopaedics,
Alpert Medical School of Brown University,
Providence, RI, USA

© Springer International Publishing AG, part of Springer Nature 2018   285
A. E. M. Eltorai et al. (eds.), *Essential Orthopedic Review*,
https://doi.org/10.1007/978-3-319-78387-1_124

(continued)

What is the most common spine deformity?	Kyphosis at the thoracolumbar junction
What is the common spine problem requiring surgery?	Spinal stenosis
What is the common skull abnormality with serious complications?	Foramen magnum stenosis
What is the key radiographic feature on an AP lumbar spine radiograph?	Narrowing of the L1–L5 interpedicular distance

Bibliography

1. Sponseller PD, Ain MC. The skeletal dysplasias. In: Weinstein SL, editor. Lovell and Winter's pediatric orthopaedics, vol. 1. 7th ed. Philadelphia: Wolters Kluwer; 2014. p. 180–6. Print.
2. Herring JA. Skeletal dysplasias. In: Herring JA, editor. Tachjian's pediatric orthopaedics: from the Texas Scottish Rite Hospital, vol. 2. 5th ed. Philadelphia: Elsevier Saunders; 2014. p. 370–85. Print.
3. Shirley ED, Ain MC. Achondroplasia: manifestations and treatment. J Am Acad Orthop Surg. 2009;17:231–41.

Chapter 125
Other Skeletal Dysplasia

Jonathan R. Schiller

What is the inheritance pattern of diastrophic dysplasia?	Autosomal recessive
Diastrophic dysplasia is a result of what defect?	Sulfate transport protein
What are the classic findings for diastrophic dysplasia?	Hitchhiker thumb and cauliflower ears

(continued)

J. R. Schiller, MD
Adolescent and Young Adult Hip Program, Orthopaedic Surgery, The Warren Alpert School of Medicine of Brown University, Providence, RI, USA

Division of Pediatric Orthopaedics and Scoliosis, Hasbro Children's Hospital, Rhode Island Hospital, Providence, RI, USA

Division of Sports Medicine, Hasbro Children's Hospital, Rhode Island Hospital, Providence, RI, USA
e-mail: jonathan_schiller@brown.edu

© Springer International Publishing AG, part of Springer Nature 2018   287
A. E. M. Eltorai et al. (eds.), *Essential Orthopedic Review*,
https://doi.org/10.1007/978-3-319-78387-1_125

(continued)

What gene defect is responsible for cleidocranial dysplasia?	RUNX 2
What bone is classically involved in cleidocranial dysplasia?	Clavicle
What is the genetic defect in campomelic dysplasia?	Sox 9
What is the inheritance pattern of campomelic dysplasia?	Autosomal dominant

Chapter 126
Chromosomal and Inherited Syndromes

Jose M. Ramirez

What is trisomy 21?	Down syndrome
What disease is associated with a deficiency in B-glucocerebrosidase?	Gaucher's disease
What is the defective protein that leads to achondroplasia?	FGR3 receptor
What is VATER?	Syndromic disorders associated with vertebral anomalies, anal atresia, tracheoesophageal fistula, esophageal atresia, and renal agenesis
What is inheritance pattern of early onset Charcot-Marie-Tooth disease?	Autosomal dominant

J. M. Ramirez, MD
Department of Orthopaedic Surgery,
Alpert Medical School of Brown University,
Providence, RI, USA

© Springer International Publishing AG, part of Springer Nature 2018   289
A. E. M. Eltorai et al. (eds.), *Essential Orthopedic Review*,
https://doi.org/10.1007/978-3-319-78387-1_126

Chapter 127
Arthritis

Jose M. Ramirez

What are the radiographic signs of arthritis?	Joint space narrowing, marginal osteophytes, subchondral sclerosis, periarticular cyst formation
True or False: Water content in collagen increases in osteoarthritis.	True
What collagen type is most commonly found in articular cartilage?	Type II (2)
What are the layers of articular cartilage?	Superficial, intermediate, deep, tidemark
What kind of cartilage is formed as a result of an injury through the tidemark?	Fibrocartilage

J. M. Ramirez, MD
Department of Orthopaedic Surgery,
Alpert Medical School of Brown University,
Providence, RI, USA

© Springer International Publishing AG, part of Springer Nature 2018   291
A. E. M. Eltorai et al. (eds.), *Essential Orthopedic Review*,
https://doi.org/10.1007/978-3-319-78387-1_127

Chapter 128
Shoulder and Elbow Deformities

Aristides I. Cruz Jr.

What percentage of the humerus' longitudinal growth comes from the proximal physis?	80%
What is the gene abnormality associated with cleidocranial dysplasia?	RUNX2/CBFA1
What form of ossification accounts for ossification of the clavicle?	Intramembranous ossification
At what age is brachial plexus birth palsy unlikely to spontaneously recover (i.e., if antigravity motor function is not displayed by age ____)?	5–6 months

(continued)

A. I. Cruz Jr., MD, MBA
Department of Orthopaedic Surgery, Warren Alpert Medical
School of Brown University, Providence, RI, USA

© Springer International Publishing AG, part of Springer Nature 2018   293
A. E. M. Eltorai et al. (eds.), *Essential Orthopedic Review*,
https://doi.org/10.1007/978-3-319-78387-1_128

(continued)

What trunk/nerve roots are most commonly involved in brachial plexus birth palsy?	Upper trunk/C5-C6
What clinical manifestations occur with chronic, upper trunk, brachial plexus birth palsy?	Shoulder abduction/external rotation weakness, internal rotation contracture, posterior glenoid deficiency/dysplasia
What is Sprengel's deformity?	It is a congenital condition of the shoulder that results in an undescended scapula which can result in abnormal motion of the shoulder
What is the most common coronal plane deformity after a supracondylar humerus fracture malunion?	Cubitus varus
What is the name of the deformity that can occur after a distal humerus lateral condyle non-union?	Fishtail deformity
What is Panner's disease?	Osteochondrosis of the capitellum
What is "Little Leaguer's Shoulder"?	Proximal humeral physiolysis resulting from overuse in an overhead throwing athlete
Avulsion fracture of the olecranon apophysis is associated with what condition?	Osteogenesis imperfecta

Chapter 129
Hand and Wrist Deformities

Aristides I. Cruz Jr.

What is Madelung's deformity?	Distal radius congenital physeal abnormality that results in distal radial growth disturbance and resultant increased distal radial inclination and volar tilt
What is "gymnast's wrist"?	Distal radial physeal repetitive stress syndrome
What is the anatomic difference between post-axial and pre-axial polydactyly?	Post-axial = ulnar sided duplication Pre-axial = radial sided duplication
What is the primary goal when surgically treating pre-axial polydactyly?	To provide a functional and stable thumb

(continued)

A. I. Cruz Jr., MD, MBA
Department of Orthopaedic Surgery, Warren Alpert Medical School of Brown University, Providence, RI, USA

© Springer International Publishing AG, part of Springer Nature 2018   295
A. E. M. Eltorai et al. (eds.), *Essential Orthopedic Review*,
https://doi.org/10.1007/978-3-319-78387-1_129

(continued)

At what age is pediatric trigger thumb unlikely to spontaneously resolve?	Two years old
What is the treatment for pediatric trigger thumb that has failed to resolve spontaneously and has failed to respond to nonoperative treatment?	A1 pulley release
What conditions are associated with radial club hand?	Thrombocytopenia absent radius (TAR) syndrome Fanconi's anemia Holt-Oram syndrome VACTERL syndrome VATER syndrome
What is clinodactyly?	Curvature of the digit in the radial-ulnar plane
What is the inheritance pattern in clinodactyly?	Autosomal dominant
What is the hand abnormality associated with Apert syndrome?	"Rosebud hand"
What is Streeter's syndrome?	Amniotic band (constriction band) syndrome
What is the difference between complex and simple syndactyly?	Simple = soft tissue involvement only Complex = bony synostosis
What classification scheme is commonly used to describe thumb duplications?	Wassel classification

Chapter 130
Genu Varum

Aristides I. Cruz Jr.

What is the name of the condition describing pathologic proximal tibia vara?	Blount's disease
What medical conditions can lead to pathologic genu varum?	Rickets, osteogenesis imperfecta, multiple epiphyseal dysplasia (MED), spondyloepiphyseal dysplasia (SED), achondroplasia, pseudoachondroplasia
What are the risk factors for pathologic tibia vara (Blount's disease)?	Early walking, obesity, African-American descent

(continued)

A. I. Cruz Jr., MD, MBA
Department of Orthopaedic Surgery, Warren Alpert Medical
School of Brown University, Providence, RI, USA

© Springer International Publishing AG, part of Springer Nature 2018   297
A. E. M. Eltorai et al. (eds.), *Essential Orthopedic Review*,
https://doi.org/10.1007/978-3-319-78387-1_130

(continued)

| Which compartment of the knee does the mechanical axis pass through in patients with genu varum? | Medial compartment |
| What is the name of the classification system commonly used to describe pathologic tibia vara? | Langenskiöld classification |

Chapter 131
Genu Valgum

Aristides I. Cruz Jr.

What is the normal amount of valgus (in degrees) at skeletal maturity?	About 5–7°
At what age is genu valgum most pronounced?	Age 3–4 years
At what age is persistent or worsening genu valgum considered pathologic?	Older than 7 years
What is "miserable malalignment"?	Excess femoral anteversion combined with excess external tibial torsion

(continued)

A. I. Cruz Jr., MD, MBA
Department of Orthopaedic Surgery, Warren Alpert Medical School of Brown University, Providence, RI, USA

© Springer International Publishing AG, part of Springer Nature 2018   299
A. E. M. Eltorai et al. (eds.), *Essential Orthopedic Review*,
https://doi.org/10.1007/978-3-319-78387-1_131

(continued)

What is Cozen's fracture?	Proximal tibial metaphyseal fracture which is associated with the development of late valgus deformity which usually resolves spontaneously
What is the treatment of choice for pathologic genu valgum in skeletally immature patients?	Temporary hemi-epiphysiodesis or "guided-growth"
Which X-ray should be ordered to diagnose and monitor genu valgum?	Bilateral, standing AP long-leg
What anatomic structure is at risk if performing a proximal tibia lateral opening wedge osteotomy to correct excess proximal tibia valgus?	Peroneal nerve
What is the normal range for the mechanical lateral distal femoral angle (mLDFA) and medial proximal tibial angle (MPTA)?	mLFDA = 87° (85–90°) MPTA = 87° (85–90°)
Which compartment of the knee does the mechanical axis pass through in patients with genu valgum?	Lateral compartment

Chapter 132
Axial Rotations

Jose M. Ramirez

What is the most common cause of intoeing in toddlers?	Internal tibial torsion
How does one measure thigh foot angle?	With the patient prone, angle formed along middle of the foot and the ipsilateral thigh
What are two additional causes of intoeing in children?	Metatarsus adductus, femoral anteversion

J. M. Ramirez, MD
Department of Orthopaedic Surgery, Alpert Medical School
of Brown University, Providence, RI, USA

© Springer International Publishing AG, part of Springer Nature 2018   301
A. E. M. Eltorai et al. (eds.), *Essential Orthopedic Review*,
https://doi.org/10.1007/978-3-319-78387-1_132

Chapter 133
Limb Deficiency

Jose M. Ramirez

What is the expected yearly contribution to longitudinal growth of the distal femoral physis/proximal tibial physis?	9 mm per year/6 mm per year
What is the expected yearly contribution to longitudinal growth of the proximal tibial physis?	6 mm per year
What is the preferred management of a patient with a 2 cm leg length discrepancy?	Observation and/or shoe lift
How is a 2–5 cm leg length discrepancy typically addressed surgically?	Epiphysiodesis of the longer extremity

J. M. Ramirez, MD
Department of Orthopaedic Surgery, Alpert Medical School
of Brown University, Providence, RI, USA

© Springer International Publishing AG, part of Springer Nature 2018   303
A. E. M. Eltorai et al. (eds.), *Essential Orthopedic Review*,
https://doi.org/10.1007/978-3-319-78387-1_133

Chapter 134
Limb Length Discrepancy

Jonathan R. Schiller

A limb length discrepancy (LLD) can be classified into what three groups?	Congenital (hemihypertrophy), dysplastic (hemimelia), acquired (trauma, tumor, infection)
What is the gold standard for accurate limb length measurement?	Radiographic assessment with limb length radiograph, scanogram, CT scanogram, EOS imaging
What is the average yearly growth of the distal femoral physis and proximal tibia physis?	9 mm, 6 mm respectively

(continued)

J. R. Schiller, MD
Adolescent and Young Adult Hip Program, The Warren Alpert
School of Medicine of Brown University, Providence, RI, USA

Division of Pediatric Orthopaedics and Scoliosis, Hasbro Children's
Hospital, Rhode Island Hospital, Providence, RI, USA

Division of Sports Medicine, Hasbro Children's Hospital,
Rhode Island Hospital, Providence, RI, USA
e-mail: jonathan_schiller@brown.edu

© Springer International Publishing AG, part of Springer Nature 2018   305
A. E. M. Eltorai et al. (eds.), *Essential Orthopedic Review*,
https://doi.org/10.1007/978-3-319-78387-1_134

(continued)

Surgery is indicated for a discrepancy of how much?	Greater than 2.5 cm
What is the treatment for discrepancies greater than 20 cm?	Amputation and prosthetic fitting
Accurate assessment for surgical timing requires what radiologic image study?	Bone age
Limb length discrepancies greater than 5 cm consists of what surgical treatment?	Contralateral epiphysiodesis with lengthening using external fixator or intramedullary device

Chapter 135
Pseudarthrosis of the Tibia

Jonathan R. Schiller

What type of bowing occurs in congenital pseudoarthrosis of the tibia?	Anterolateral
Congenital pseudarthrosis of the tibia is associated with what underlying pathology?	Neurofibromatosis type 1, 50%
What is the goal of treatment for anterolateral bowing of the tibia?	To prevent fracture
What is the treatment for anterolateral bowing to prevent fracture?	Bracing

(continued)

J. R. Schiller, MD
Adolescent and Young Adult Hip Program, The Warren Alpert
School of Medicine of Brown University, Providence, RI, USA

Division of Pediatric Orthopaedics and Scoliosis, Hasbro Children's
Hospital, Rhode Island Hospital, Providence, RI, USA

Division of Sports Medicine, Hasbro Children's Hospital,
Rhode Island Hospital, Providence, RI, USA
e-mail: jonathan_schiller@brown.edu

© Springer International Publishing AG, part of Springer Nature 2018   307
A. E. M. Eltorai et al. (eds.), *Essential Orthopedic Review*,
https://doi.org/10.1007/978-3-319-78387-1_135

(continued)

What is the treatment for fracture of the anterolateral bowing of the tibia?	Operative fixation with Ilizarov or intramedullary fixation
Failure to achieve union in a pseudarthrosis of the tibia may require what procedure?	Below-knee amputation

Chapter 136
Foot and Ankle Deformities

Jonathan R. Schiller

What are the characteristics of a congenital vertical talus (CVT)?	Rigid rocker bottom deformity, fixed dorsal dislocation of talonavicular joint
What neuromuscular disorder is often associated with CVT?	Myelomeningocele
What test is diagnostic for CVT?	Forced plantar flexion on lateral radiograph of foot
What is the most common congenital foot disorder?	Clubfoot

(continued)

J. R. Schiller, MD
Adolescent and Young Adult Hip Program, The Warren Alpert
School of Medicine of Brown University, Providence, RI, USA

Division of Pediatric Orthopaedics and Scoliosis, Hasbro Children's
Hospital, Rhode Island Hospital, Providence, RI, USA

Division of Sports Medicine, Hasbro Children's Hospital, Rhode
Island Hospital, Providence, RI, USA
e-mail: jonathan_schiller@brown.edu

© Springer International Publishing AG, part of Springer Nature 2018   309
A. E. M. Eltorai et al. (eds.), *Essential Orthopedic Review*,
https://doi.org/10.1007/978-3-319-78387-1_136

(continued)

What are the characteristics of a clubfoot?	Midfoot cavus, forefoot adductus, hindfoot varus, and equinus
What is the gold standard of clubfoot treatment?	Ponseti casting
What is the order of correction for a clubfoot using the Ponseti casting method?	CAVE; cavus, adductus, varus, equinus
What is a bean-shaped foot deformity otherwise known as?	Metatarsus adductus
What is the primary treatment of metatarsus adductus?	Observation/stretching
What is a tarsal coalition?	Abnormal connection between two bones in the midfoot or hindfoot
What types of coalitions can occur?	Osseous, cartilaginous, or fibrous
A coalition is often present with what type of foot?	Rigid flat foot with minimal subtalar motion
What imaging study is preferred for the diagnosis of a tarsal coalition?	CT scan
What are the two most common coalitions?	Calcaneal navicular, talocalcaneal
What characterizes a cavovarus foot?	Elevated medial arch, plantar flexion of the first ray, hindfoot varus
This deformity is often associated with what neuromuscular or spinal cord problems?	Charcot-Marie-Tooth disease, tethered cord
What test is used to distinguish a flexible hindfoot?	Coleman block test
Hindfoot varus is driven by what deformity?	Forefoot plantar flexion of the first ray

Chapter 137
Idiopathic Scoliosis

Daniel Brian Carlin Reid

Which is more common: right or left thoracic curve?	Right thoracic curve
Define the Cobb angle.	On PA radiograph: angle of intersection between a line drawn parallel to the superior endplate of the superior end vertebra and a line parallel to the inferior endplate of the inferior end vertebra of a curve deformity
Name indications for MRI scan prior to operative treatment of patients with scoliosis.	Atypical curve pattern (e.g., left thoracic curve), rapid curve progression, painful scoliosis, neurologic signs/symptoms, asymmetric abdominal reflex, apical kyphosis of the thoracic curve, juvenile-onset scoliosis, associated syndrome, or congenital abnormalities

(continued)

D. B. C. Reid, MD, MPH
Department of Orthopaedics, Rhode Island Hospital, Brown University, Providence, RI, USA

© Springer International Publishing AG, part of Springer Nature 2018   311
A. E. M. Eltorai et al. (eds.), *Essential Orthopedic Review*,
https://doi.org/10.1007/978-3-319-78387-1_137

(continued)

What are the commonly cited Cobb angle cutoffs for different idiopathic scoliosis treatment modalities?	<25°: observation, 25–45°: bracing, >45–50°: operative treatment
What is the goal of bracing?	To stop or slow curve progression
What is the unique risk of posterior fusion alone in skeletally immature patients?	Crankshaft phenomenon (anterior spine continues to grow after posterior fusion, increasing rotation/deformity)

Chapter 138
Neuromuscular Scoliosis

Daniel Brian Carlin Reid

Name some major ways in which neuromuscular scoliosis is different than idiopathic	More rapidly progressive, can progress after skeletal maturity, associated with pelvic obliquity, often longer curves involving more vertebrae, higher rate of pulmonary complications
In general, has bracing generally been proven to improve deformity or slow progression of disease in patients with neuromuscular scoliosis?	No

(continued)

D. B. C. Reid, MD, MPH
Department of Orthopaedics, Rhode Island Hospital,
Brown University, Providence, RI, USA

© Springer International Publishing AG, part of Springer Nature 2018   313
A. E. M. Eltorai et al. (eds.), *Essential Orthopedic Review*,
https://doi.org/10.1007/978-3-319-78387-1_138

(continued)

Name common underlying conditions resulting in neuromuscular scoliosis	Cerebral palsy, Rett syndrome, muscular dystrophy, Friedreich's Ataxia, spina bifida, spinal muscular atrophy, neurofibromatosis, arthrogryposis, polio, traumatic paralysis
Why is nutritional status important to the orthopedic surgeon treating patients with neuromuscular scoliosis?	Poor nutritional status is associated with increased overall complications (infection, longer intubations, longer hospital stays, etc.)
What nutritional markers have been associated with increased wound complications?	Albumin <3.5 g/dL, WBC <1500 Leukocytes/μL

Chapter 139
Congenital Spinal Anomalies

Daniel Brian Carlin Reid

Congenital scoliosis is generally caused by an error in normal fetal development during what time period?	Fourth–sixth week of gestation
What is the most common inheritance pattern of congenital scoliosis?	Spontaneous
Name some known maternal exposures associated with congenital scoliosis	Alcohol, valproic acid, hyperthermia, diabetes
What is VACTERL association?	Known association between vertebral anomolies, anal atresia, cardiac anomolies, tracheo-esophageal fistula, renal anomalies, and limb defects

(continued)

D. B. C. Reid, MD, MPH
Department of Orthopaedics, Rhode Island Hospital,
Brown University, Providence, RI, USA

© Springer International Publishing AG, part of Springer Nature 2018   315
A. E. M. Eltorai et al. (eds.), *Essential Orthopedic Review*,
https://doi.org/10.1007/978-3-319-78387-1_139

(continued)

Which patients with congenital scoliosis require MRI before surgery?	All patients, to evaluate for intraspinal abnormalities
What are the three basic types of defects in congenital scoliosis?	Failure of formation, failure of segmentation, mixed
What congenital defect confers the lowest risk of progression of congenital scoliosis?	Block vertebrae
What congenital defect confers the highest risk of progression of congenital scoliosis?	Unilateral unsegmented bar with contralateral hemivertebrae

Chapter 140
Scheuermann's Kyphosis

Daniel Brian Carlin Reid

What is considered normal range for thoracic kyphosis?	20–45°
How is Scheuermann's kyphosis defined?	Rigid thoracic kyphosis >45° with >5° anterior wedging at three consecutive vertebrae
Does Scheurmann's kyphosis correct to normal with hyperextension?	No
What are other common radiographic findings in patients with Scheurmann's kyphosis?	Compensatory lumbar hyperlordosis, spondylolysis, scoliosis, disc space narrowing, end plate changes, Schmorl nodes
What degree of kyphosis is often cited as an indication for surgery?	>75°

D. B. C. Reid, MD, MPH
Department of Orthopaedics, Rhode Island Hospital,
Brown University, Providence, RI, USA

© Springer International Publishing AG, part of Springer Nature 2018   317
A. E. M. Eltorai et al. (eds.), *Essential Orthopedic Review*,
https://doi.org/10.1007/978-3-319-78387-1_140

Chapter 141
Cervical Spine Disorders (Pediatric)

Daniel Brian Carlin Reid

What pediatric syndrome is characterized by abnormalities in multiple cervical segments caused by failure of normal segmentation?	Klippel-Feil syndrome
Why do patients with trisomy 21 often get cervical spine flexion-extension views prior to elective surgery?	To evaluate for atlantoaxial instability prior to intubation
What study is considered the gold standard for diagnosing rotary atlantoaxial subluxation?	Dynamic CT
What is the name of the condition in which a patient is diagnosed with rotary atlantoaxial subluxation after recent retropharyngeal abscess or respiratory infection?	Grisel's disease

(continued)

D. B. C. Reid, MD, MPH
Department of Orthopaedics, Rhode Island Hospital,
Brown University, Providence, RI, USA

© Springer International Publishing AG, part of Springer Nature 2018   319
A. E. M. Eltorai et al. (eds.), *Essential Orthopedic Review*,
https://doi.org/10.1007/978-3-319-78387-1_141

(continued)

What structure limits anterior translation of C1 (atlas) on C2 (axis)?	Transverse ligament
What anatomic variant of C2 is often mistaken for an odontoid fracture?	Os odontoideum
What study can help differentiate pediatric cervical spine pseudosubluxation from true injury?	Flexion-extension X-rays (pseudosubluxaton will reduce on extension films)
What is it called when the odontoid migrates into the foramen magnum, potentially impinging on the brainstem?	Basilar invagination
What advanced imaging study can be used to indirectly visualize neural elements and/or spinal cord compression in patients who cannot undergo an MRI	CT myelogram

Chapter 142
Spondylolysis and Spondylolisthesis

Daniel Brian Carlin Reid

Spondylolysis refers to a defect or fracture of which structure?	Pars interarticularis
How is spondylolisthesis defined?	Anterior translation of one vertebra on the vertebra below it (most commonly L5 on S1)
What is spondyloptosis?	Greater than 100% slip of one vertebral body on the once below it (Meyerding Grade 5 slip)
Which X-ray views show the "scottie dog"?	Oblique radiographs
What type of spondylolisthesis is most common in adolescents?	Isthmic

(continued)

D. B. C. Reid, MD, MPH
Department of Orthopaedics, Rhode Island Hospital,
Brown University, Providence, RI, USA

© Springer International Publishing AG, part of Springer Nature 2018   321
A. E. M. Eltorai et al. (eds.), *Essential Orthopedic Review*,
https://doi.org/10.1007/978-3-319-78387-1_142

(continued)

What nerve root is most commonly affected by L5-S1 isthmic spondylolisthesis?	L5
What is the main structure at risk with attempted reduction of L5-S1 spondylolisthesis?	L5 nerve root

Chapter 143
Spine Injuries

Daniel Brian Carlin Reid

What physical exam finding signals the end of spinal shock?	Return of bulbocavernosus reflex
What vital sign is most helpful in differentiation neurogenic shock from hypovolemic shock?	Pulse (neurogenic shock results in relative bradycardia in setting of hypotension)
How does the American spinal injury association (ASIA) classification define the neurologic level of injury?	The most caudal segment of spinal cord with normal sensory and at least 3/5 (antigravity) motor function on both sides of the body
Why are cervical spine injuries more common in children <8 years old?	Large head-to-body-ratio

(continued)

D. B. C. Reid, MD, MPH
Department of Orthopaedics, Rhode Island Hospital,
Brown University, Providence, RI, USA

© Springer International Publishing AG, part of Springer Nature 2018   323
A. E. M. Eltorai et al. (eds.), *Essential Orthopedic Review*,
https://doi.org/10.1007/978-3-319-78387-1_143

(continued)

What three X-ray views are most commonly used to evaluate the cervical spine in pediatric patients following trauma?	Anteroposterior (AP), lateral, open-mouth odontoid
Where do odontoid fractures commonly occur in children?	Through the synchondrosis (Salter-Harris type 1 injury)

Part VI
Systemic Conditions

Chapter 144
Septic Arthritis

Stephen Marcaccio

Define septic arthritis.	A serious orthopedic condition characterized by infection of synovial joints resulting in rapid destruction of articular cartilage
What are three mechanisms of joint infection?	1. Bacteremia 2. Direct inoculation 3. Contiguous spread (adjacent osteomyelitis)
What organism is the most common cause of septic arthritis?	Staph aureus
What is the classic presentation for Neisseria septic arthritis?	Young sexually active adolescents and young adults

(continued)

S. Marcaccio, MD
Department of Orthopaedic Surgery, Rhode Island Hospital, Brown University, Providence, RI, USA
e-mail: stephen_marcaccio@brown.edu

© Springer International Publishing AG, part of Springer Nature 2018   327
A. E. M. Eltorai et al. (eds.), *Essential Orthopedic Review*,
https://doi.org/10.1007/978-3-319-78387-1_144

(continued)

What types of patients typically present with SC joint infections?	IV drug users
How do patients usually present with septic arthritis?	Pain in joint area, fevers (60% cases), joint resting in position that allows maximum joint volume (FABER for hip). Warm and tender to the touch, inability to bear weight, no ROM
What is the classic workup for suspected septic arthritis?	ESR, CRP, WBC, aspirate the joint fluid
What is the definitive treatment for septic arthritis?	This is an orthopedic emergency: IV abx, operative irrigation and debridement and drainage of the joint is essential

Chapter 145
Osteomyelitis

Adam Driesman

What is the most common organism found in osteomyelitis of adults?	Staph aureus
What is the most common organism found in sickle cell patients with osteomyelitis?	Still Staph aureus, while Salmonella species is pathognomonic
What is the most common transmission of osteomyelitis in the pediatric population?	Hematogenous seeding, typically to the metaphyseal region

(continued)

A. Driesman, MD
Department of Orthopaedics, NYU Hospital for Joint Diseases, New York, NY, USA

Drs. Ramirez and Terek are at associated with Brown University, Providence, RI, USA
e-mail: adam_driesman@brown.edu

© Springer International Publishing AG, part of Springer Nature 2018   329
A. E. M. Eltorai et al. (eds.), *Essential Orthopedic Review*,
https://doi.org/10.1007/978-3-319-78387-1_145

(continued)

What is the name of a common classification scheme for chronic osteomyelitis?	Cierny and Mader classification
What are the four stages of this classification to describe anatomic location?	Stage 1: Medullary Stage 2: Superficial Stage 3: Localized Stage 4: Diffuse
What are the three types of this classification to describe the patient's immune status?	Type A: Normal Type B: Compromised Type C: Treatment is worse to patient than infection
What is a sequestrum?	Necrotic bone that can serve as a source for infection in chronic osteomyelitis. It is typically sclerotic and avascular, thereby limiting antibiotic penetration
What is the name of new bone formation that occurs as a periosteal reaction to chronic osteomyelitis?	Involucrum
What inflammatory markers are elevated in chronic osteomyelitis?	ESR and CRP WBC is only elevated in 35% of cases
What is the gold standard in diagnosis?	Biopsy specimen for evaluation of histology and microbiology
Formation of what makes peri-implant infection difficult to treat?	Biofilm

Chapter 146
Necrotizing Fasciitis

Adam Driesman

What is the predominant bacteria that causes necrotizing fasciitis?	Non-group A streptococci
What are more common, monomicrobial or polymicrobial infections?	Polymicrobial infections
What patient risk factors predispose patients to necrotizing fasciitis?	Immunosuppressed (AIDS/chemo), DM, PVD, alcoholism, IV drug use
What is the typical clinical course of this infection?	Rapid progression that requires emergent treatment

(continued)

A. Driesman, MD
Department of Orthopaedics, NYU Langone Orthopedic Hospital, New York, NY, USA

Drs. Ramirez and Terek are at associated with Brown University, Providence, RI, USA
e-mail: adam_driesman@brown.edu

© Springer International Publishing AG, part of Springer Nature 2018   331
A. E. M. Eltorai et al. (eds.), *Essential Orthopedic Review*,
https://doi.org/10.1007/978-3-319-78387-1_146

(continued)

What are some of the clinical physical exam signs?	Skin abscess, bullae, blue discoloration, pain, swelling, non-pitting edema In comparison, gas gangrene typically described as pus that is "dish-water soap" like appearance
What is the main origin of infection?	Minimal trauma or minor skin lesions Note: can still occur in the absence of trauma
What is the mainstay of treatment?	Early surgical debridement and wide-spectrum antibiotic therapy
What is the mortality rate found in these patients?	Upwards of 30%

Chapter 147
Osteoarthritis

Sean Esmende and Hardeep Singh

What are the primary components of articular (hyaline) cartilage?	1. Extracellular matrix (90% collagen and proteoglycan) 2. Chondrocytes 3. Water
How does water content differ between normal aging and osteoarthritis?	Water decreases with normal aging and decreases with osteoarthritis
What are the zones of articular cartilage?	1. Superficial zone 2. Intermediate zone 3. Deep (basal) later 4. Tidemark 5. Subchondral bone

(continued)

S. Esmende, MD (✉)
Orthopedic Associates of Hartford, Division of Spine Surgery,
The Bone and Joint Institute, Hartford Hospital,
Hartford, CT, USA

H. Singh, MD
Department of Orthopaedic Surgery, New England
Musculoskeletal Institute, University of Connecticut School
of Medicine, Farmington, CT, USA

© Springer International Publishing AG, part of Springer Nature 2018   333
A. E. M. Eltorai et al. (eds.), *Essential Orthopedic Review*,
https://doi.org/10.1007/978-3-319-78387-1_147

(continued)

What effect does immobilization have on cartilage?	Leads to cartilage thinning and proteoglycan loss
With aging, what happens to chondrocyte size and the ratio of keratin sulfate to chondroitin sulfate?	– Increase in chondrocyte size – Increase in keratin sulfate to chondroitin sulfate
What effect does moderate repetitive loading have on cartilage and proteoglycans?	Moderate running increases cartilage thickness and proteoglycan content
How is cartilage nourished?	– Synovial fluid at the cartilage surface – Subchondral bone at the base
What are the different forms of lubrication?	1. Elastohydrodynamic 2. Boundary (slippery surface) 3. Boosted (fluid entrapment) 4. Hydrodynamic 5. Weeping
What is the difference in cartilage healing between a deep and superficial laceration?	– Deep laceration leads to fibrocartilage healing – Superficial laceration leads to chondrocyte proliferation with NO healing

Chapter 148
Rheumatoid Arthritis

Stuart T. Schwartz

What is the inflammatory erosive synovial tissue in rheumatoid arthritis?	The **pannus**
Name two hand deformities in rheumatoid arthritis.	**Swan neck** and **boutonniere deformities**
Which joints in the hands are spared from synovitis in rheumatoid arthritis?	DIP joints
What condition should be excluded before surgical intubation in rheumatoid arthritis patients?	C1–C2 subluxation
What are two diagnostic serologies found in rheumatoid arthritis?	**Rheumatoid factor** and **anti-cyclic citrullinated peptide antibodies**

(continued)

S. T. Schwartz, MD
Alpert Medical School of Brown University, Providence, RI, USA
e-mail: sschwartz@lifespan.org

© Springer International Publishing AG, part of Springer Nature 2018   335
A. E. M. Eltorai et al. (eds.), *Essential Orthopedic Review*,
https://doi.org/10.1007/978-3-319-78387-1_148

(continued)

What is the name of the syndrome in patients with rheumatoid arthritis associated with splenomegaly and leukopenia (specifically, neutropenia)?	**Felty's syndrome**
What is the name of subcutaneous nodules found on the extensor surfaces and hands of patients with rheumatoid arthritis?	**Rheumatoid nodules**

Chapter 149
Crystal-Induced Arthropathy

James Levins

What type of birefringence are gout crystals?	Negative, yellow when parallel to direction of polarization, needle-shaped
What is the mainstay of medical treatment for an acute gout attack?	NSAIDs or colchicine, if chronic kidney disease (CKD) then steroids
What surgical emergency has to be in your differential for an acute gout attack?	Septic arthritis—patients with crystalline arthropathy are also at increased risk for developing septic arthritis
What is the typical white blood cell (WBC) range in crystalline arthropathy?	2000–50,000 WBC, neutrophil predominant

(continued)

J. Levins, MD
Department of Orthopaedic Surgery, Brown University,
Providence, RI, USA

© Springer International Publishing AG, part of Springer Nature 2018   337
A. E. M. Eltorai et al. (eds.), *Essential Orthopedic Review*,
https://doi.org/10.1007/978-3-319-78387-1_149

(continued)

In patients with calcium pyrophosphate deposition disease (pseudogout), what is a common finding on radiographs of the affected joint?	Chondrocalcinosis (calcification of cartilage)

Chapter 150
Fibromyalgia

Deepan Dalal and Pieusha Malhotra

What are the cardinal symptoms of fibromyalgia?	Diffuse pain, fatigue, lack of refreshing sleep, cognitive symptoms (memory, concentration)
Who is typically affected by fibromyalgia?	Younger (20–55 years) female
What is the pathophysiology of fibromyalgia?	Amplified pain perception resulting from central sensitization

(continued)

D. Dalal, MD, MPH (✉)
Department of Medicine-Rheumatology, Brown University, Providence, RI, USA

P. Malhotra, MD, MPH
Department of Medicine-Rheumatology, Roger Williams Medical Center, Providence, RI, USA

© Springer International Publishing AG, part of Springer Nature 2018   339
A. E. M. Eltorai et al. (eds.), *Essential Orthopedic Review*,
https://doi.org/10.1007/978-3-319-78387-1_150

(continued)

What are the commonly associated symptoms with fibromyalgia?	Symptoms of irritable bowel syndrome, interstitial cystitis, headaches/migraines, premenstrual syndrome, depression/anxiety, and host of other somatic manifestations
What tests are performed for diagnosis of fibromyalgia?	Clinical diagnosis, inflammatory markers are normal, serologies (RF, ANA) are often unremarkable
In addition to the above, what diseases should be ruled out?	Primary sleep disorders like sleep apnea, restless leg syndrome
What are the non-pharmacologic interventions for fibromyalgia?	(1) Aerobic exercise, (2) Cognitive behavioral therapy, (3) Evaluation of and correction of sleep disorders (CPAP machine, etc.) and (4) Complementary/alternative medicine (yoga, Tai-chi, acupuncture)
What are the drugs approved for treatment of fibromyalgia?	Initial therapy with Amitriptyline (or even Cyclobenzaprine) followed by Duloxetine/Milnacipran/Gabapentin. Other drugs to consider acetaminophen, tramadol, and SSRIs. NSAIDs do not work very well

Chapter 151
Seronegative Spondyloarthropathies

Eren O. Kuris

What are seronegative spondyloarthropathies?	Systemic rheumatologic disorders of the axial skeleton
Why are they considered to be seronegative?	Because blood tests are traditionally negative for rheumatoid factor, which is a marker that can detect many rheumatological conditions
What are some common examples of seronegative spondyloarthropathies?	Ankylosing spondylitis
	Reactive arthritis
	Psoriatic arthritis
	Juvenile idiopathic arthritis
	Enteropathic arthritis

(continued)

E. O. Kuris, MD
Department of Orthopaedic Surgery, Warren Alpert Medical School of Brown University, Providence, RI, USA

© Springer International Publishing AG, part of Springer Nature 2018   341
A. E. M. Eltorai et al. (eds.), *Essential Orthopedic Review*,
https://doi.org/10.1007/978-3-319-78387-1_151

(continued)

What genetic marker is frequently associated with seronegative spondyloarthropathies?	Human Leukocyte Antigen B27 (HLA-B27)
What are some common manifestations of these conditions?	Sacroiliitis Uveitis Inflammatory joint arthritis Enthesitis
What radiographic spine features are associated with ankylosing spondylitis?	Calcifications of the intervertebral discs and ligamentous complexes (syndesmophytes) Ankylosis of the facet joints ("bamboo spine")
What is the gold standard for treatment of these conditions?	Biologic drugs, such as disease-modifying antirheumatic drugs (DMARDs) For example, antitumor necrosis factor-α inhibitors

Suggested Reading

1. Herkowitz HN, Garfin SR, Eismont FJ, Bel GR, Balderston RA. Rothman-Simeone The spine. 6th ed. Philadelphia, PA: Saunders; 2011
2. Khalessi AA, Oh BC, Wang MY. Medical management of ankylosing spondylitis. Neurosurg Focus. 2008;24(1):E4. https://doi.org/10.3171/FOC/2008/24/1/E4. Review. PubMed PMID: 18290742.
3. Kubiak EN, Moskovich R, Errico TJ, Di Cesare PE. Orthopaedic management of ankylosing spondylitis. J Am Acad Orthop Surg. 2005;13(4):267–78. PubMed PMID: 16112983.

Chapter 152
Polymyalgia Rheumatica

Tina Brar and Joanne Szczygiel Cunha

What are the symptoms of polymyalgia rheumatica (PMR)?	Pain and stiffness in the proximal muscles of the shoulders and/or pelvic girdle
Which population does PMR affect?	Patients aged > 50 years, with average age of onset of about 70 years. Caucasians are largely affected with a female predominance
What are the usual laboratory findings?	Elevated erythrocyte sedimentation rate (ESR), often >100 mm/h is the characteristic laboratory finding. But can occur with normal or mildly elevated ESR (>40 mm/h). C-reactive protein (CRP) is also usually elevated

(continued)

T. Brar, MD (✉) · J. S. Cunha, MD
Division of Rheumatology, The Warren Alpert School of Medicine of Brown University, Providence, RI, USA
e-mail: joanne_szczygiel@brown.edu

© Springer International Publishing AG, part of Springer Nature 2018   343
A. E. M. Eltorai et al. (eds.), *Essential Orthopedic Review*,
https://doi.org/10.1007/978-3-319-78387-1_152

(continued)

What other rheumatologic disease is PMR related to?	Giant cell arteritis (GCA). In patients with PMR, giant cell arteritis may occur in 30% of these patients. While in patients with GCA, polymyalgia rheumatica may occur in 40–60% of these individuals
What are some symptoms of giant cell arteritis?	New onset headache, jaw claudication, scalp tenderness, and visual changes (i.e., vision loss)
What is the main treatment of PMR?	Oral glucocorticoids. Prednisone is usually given at starting doses of 10–20 mg per day. Usually rapid improvement in patients' symptoms is seen in 1–2 days
What is the usually course of PMR?	Steroids are slowly tapered over months to year(s) based on patient's clinical response
What is the treatment for suspected giant cell arteritis?	Higher doses of steroids should be started immediately especially in patients with progressive symptoms or visual loss

Chapter 153
Osteoporosis

James Levins

What T-score is diagnostic for osteoporosis?	Less than −2.5
How do bisphosphonates work?	Increase osteoclast apoptosis, which inhibits bone resorption
Why is it recommended that patients stop taking bisphosphonates after 5 years?	Increased incidence of atypical subtrochanteric fracture
What are the radiographic findings of an atypical bisphosphonate subtrochanteric fracture?	Lateral cortical thickening, medial spike, transverse fracture line

(continued)

J. Levins, MD
Department of Orthopaedic Surgery, Brown University,
Providence, RI, USA

© Springer International Publishing AG, part of Springer Nature 2018   345
A. E. M. Eltorai et al. (eds.), *Essential Orthopedic Review*,
https://doi.org/10.1007/978-3-319-78387-1_153

(continued)

What are the most common fragility fractures?	Vertebral compression fracture, hip fracture (intertrochanteric or femoral neck), distal radius fracture, proximal humerus fracture
Are locking or nonlocking plates typically used in osteoporotic bone?	Locking plates—secondary to poor cortical bone stock, locking plates provide a more rigid construct to augment fixation
In the general population of those age > 60 years old, what is the 1-year mortality after a low-energy hip fracture?	Approximately 20–30%, with rates up to 50% in high-risk populations [1]

References

1. Schnell S, Friedman SM, Mendelson DA, Bingham KW, Kates SL. The 1-year mortality of patients treated in a hip fracture program for elders. Geriatr Orthop Surg Rehabil. 2010;1(1):6–14. https://doi.org/10.1177/2151458510378105.

Chapter 154
Rickets and Osteomalacia Review

Jeanne Delgado

Without mineralization due to low calcium, ossification of ___ to ___ fails	Cartilage, bone
At the end of long bones, these are open with rickets, but closed in those with osteomalacia	Epiphyseal growth plates
Deficiency in any of these three can cause rickets or osteomalacia.	Calcium, vitamin D, phosphate
Which organ converts vitamin D into its active form $1\text{--}25(OH)_2$?	Kidney
Vitamin D (increases/decreases) Ca^{2+} and (increases/decreases) PO_4^{3-}	Increases, increases

(continued)

J. Delgado, MD
Children's National Medical Center, Washington, DC, USA

© Springer International Publishing AG, part of Springer Nature 2018   347
A. E. M. Eltorai et al. (eds.), *Essential Orthopedic Review*,
https://doi.org/10.1007/978-3-319-78387-1_154

(continued)

Parathyroid hormone (increases/decreases) Ca^{2+} and (increases/decreases) PO_4^{3-}	Increases, decreases
What are the top risk factors for rickets?	Breastfeeding without vitamin supplementation, darkly pigmented skin, cities in northern latitude
Characteristic of rickets, rachitic rosary is often seen on which radiographic study?	Chest X-ray
Rickets can cause what spinal abnormalities?	Scoliosis, kyphosis, lordosis
With rickets, which portion of long bone appears widened, cupped, frayed, or even invisible on radiograph?	Metaphyses
What is often the first clinical presentation of osteomalacia?	Acute fracture
Name other subtle symptoms of osteomalacia.	Low back pain, bone pain, muscle pain, hypotonia

Chapter 155
Chronic Kidney Disease-Mineral and Bone Disorder: "Renal Osteodystrophy"

Janake Patel and Laura Amorese-O'Connell

What are the three components of CKD-MBD?	1. Disorders of calcium, phosphorous, parathyroid hormone (PTH), fibroblast growth factor 23 (FGF23), and vitamin D metabolism 2. Derangements of bone turnover, mineralization, volume linear growth, or strength 3. Extraskeletal calcification

(continued)

J. Patel, MD
Roger William Medical Center, Boston University,
Boston, MA, USA

L. Amorese-O'Connell, MD (✉)
The Warren Alpert Medical School of Brown University,
Providence, RI, USA
e-mail: laura.amorese-o'connell@va.gov

© Springer International Publishing AG, part of Springer Nature 2018   349
A. E. M. Eltorai et al. (eds.), *Essential Orthopedic Review*,
https://doi.org/10.1007/978-3-319-78387-1_155

(continued)

What is "renal osteodystrophy"?	Term exclusive for bone morphology derangements associated to chronic kidney disease
What are the systems involved in the pathophysiology of CKD-MBD?	Kidney, bone, intestine, and vasculature
What is the glomerular filtration rate (GFR) at which most components of CKD-MBD are already present?	40 mL/min or below
What is the earliest stage of chronic kidney disease at which bone disease can be observed?	CKD stage 2 (estimated GFR 60–89 mL/min/1.73 m^2)
What is a major feature of CKD-MBD?	Secondary hyperparathyroidism
What is secondary hyperparathyroidism?	Persistently increased PTH secondary to: Increased phosphate and FGF23 concentration in serum Decreased calcium and vitamin D (calcitriol) level in serum Reduced vitamin D receptors, calcium-sensing receptors, fibroblast growth factor receptors, and Klotho in parathyroid gland cells
What is the intervention for definitive diagnosis of "renal osteodystrophy"?	Bone biopsy

Chapter 156
Paget's Disease of the Bone

Janake Patel and Laura Amorese-O'Connell

What is the most common clinical presentation of Paget's disease of the bone (PDB)?	Asymptomatic disease with incidental finding of elevated serum alkaline phosphatase of bone origin
What is the most common symptom of Paget's disease?	Bone pain
What is the typical atraumatic fracture of long bone in Paget's patients?	Transverse or "Chalk-stick" (not spiral) fracture
What type of bone lesions are seen on plain radiographs?	Osteolytic, osteoblastic, and mixed lesions

(continued)

J. Patel, MD
Roger William Medical Center, Boston University,
Providence, RI, USA

L. Amorese-O'Connell, MD (✉)
The Warren Alpert Medical School of Brown University,
Providence, RI, USA
e-mail: laura.amorese-o'connell@va.gov

© Springer International Publishing AG, part of Springer Nature 2018
A. E. M. Eltorai et al. (eds.), *Essential Orthopedic Review*,
https://doi.org/10.1007/978-3-319-78387-1_156

(continued)

What is the treatment of choice for Paget's disease of the bone?	Bisphosphonates
How many weeks do you treat in an individual with PDB before scheduled orthopedic surgery?	Minimum 6 weeks
What is the most commonly involved joint in monostatic (single site) disease?	Pelvis
What causes excessive bleeding during orthopedic surgery in patients with Paget's disease of the bone?	Highly vascular stromal tissue replacing normal bone marrow
What other imaging modality besides plain films can be utilized for the diagnoses of Paget's disease of the bone?	Bone scan
What is the most common neurologic complication of Paget's?	Deafness

Chapter 157
Systemic Lupus Erythematosus

Tina Brar and Joanne Szczygiel Cunha

What is systemic lupus erythematosus (SLE)?	Chronic disease characterized by immune system dysfunction leading to autoantibody formation and immune complex deposition causing organ injury
SLE predominantly affects which population?	Women of child-bearing age (15–45 years), more commonly affecting non-Caucasian persons
What is the most common antibody found in SLE?	Anti-nuclear antigen (ANA), seen in >95% of SLE patients
Which antibodies are highly specific for renal disease?	Anti-double-stranded DNA antibody (anti-dsDNA) and anti-Sm antibodies

(continued)

T. Brar, MD (✉) · J. S. Cunha, MD
Division of Rheumatology, The Warren Alpert School of Medicine of Brown University, Providence, RI, USA
e-mail: joanne_szczygiel@brown.edu

© Springer International Publishing AG, part of Springer Nature 2018   353
A. E. M. Eltorai et al. (eds.), *Essential Orthopedic Review*,
https://doi.org/10.1007/978-3-319-78387-1_157

(continued)

In pregnant SLE patients, which maternal antibodies can help identify pregnancies at risk for neonatal lupus syndrome?	Anti-SSa (Rho) and anti-SSb (La)
What is the antibody that is associated with drug-induced lupus, which is reversible on stopping the offending medication?	Anti-histone antibody
What is the most characteristic lupus rash?	Malar rash—erythematous rash over the malar prominences and nasal bridge that spares the nasolabial folds
Which antibodies can help identify SLE patients at risk for a hypercoagulable state?	Antiphospholipid antibodies: Lupus anticoagulant, anti-β_2 glycoprotein-I, and anti-cardiolipin antibodies
SLE patients have a variable, relapsing-remitting course; acute flares of the disease and severe life-threatening complications need to be treated with?	Corticosteroids, typically oral doses but higher intravenous doses are used in severe, life-threatening situations
Which medication is the cornerstone of SLE therapy, which helps reduce flares and prevent organ damage, decreases thrombosis risk, and improves survival of patients?	Hydroxychloroquine

Chapter 158
Osteonecrosis

Deepan Dalal and Pieusha Malhotra

Which drugs are most commonly associated with osteonecrosis?	Glucocorticoids and alcohol
Which medical condition increases the risk of getting osteonecrosis?	Trauma, lupus, antiphospholipid syndrome, decompression sickness, sickle cell disease, Gaucher's disease
Which is the most common site of osteonecrosis?	Femoral head, femoral condyles, tibial plateaus, small bones of hand and foot

(continued)

D. Dalal, MD, MPH (✉)
Department of Medicine-Rheumatology, Brown University,
Providence, RI, USA

P. Malhotra, MD, MPH
Department of Medicine-Rheumatology, Roger Williams Medical
Center, Providence, RI, USA

© Springer International Publishing AG, part of Springer Nature 2018   355
A. E. M. Eltorai et al. (eds.), *Essential Orthopedic Review*,
https://doi.org/10.1007/978-3-319-78387-1_158

(continued)

Which is the most sensitive test to diagnose symptomatic osteonecrosis?	MRI (Other tests used—Tc-99 Bone scan)
What is the pathognomonic sign on X-ray?	Crescent sign
What is the differential diagnosis of osteonecrosis?	Consider diagnosis of primary bone marrow edema syndrome—also called transient osteoporosis of hip (TOH), spontaneous osteonecrosis of knee (SONK), (causalgia, reflex sympathetic dystrophy, complex regional pain syndrome) [better evaluated with bone scan]
Besides pain control and reduction of weight bearing, what other drugs can be considered for osteonecrosis?	Bisphosphonates, statins, anticoagulants, and vasodilators like iloprost
What are the surgical treatment options?	Core decompression, bone graft, osteotomy, and joint replacement

Chapter 159
Benign Bone Tumors

Jose M. Ramirez, Adam Driesman, and Richard Terek

What population is most likely to form an osteoid osteoma?	Young males in the second or third decade of life?
What is the typical presentation of an osteoid osteoma?	Pain that is worse at night. Pain will improve with use of NSAIDs

(continued)

J. M. Ramirez, MD (✉)
Department of Orthopaedic Surgery, Alpert Medical School, Brown University, Providence, RI, USA

A. Driesman, MD
Department of Orthopaedics, NYU Langone Orthopedic Hospital, New York, NY, USA

Drs. Ramirez and Terek are at associated with Brown University, Providence, RI, USA
e-mail: adam_driesman@brown.edu

R. Terek, MD
Warren Alpert Medical School of Brown University, Providence, RI, USA
e-mail: richard_terek@brown.edu

© Springer International Publishing AG, part of Springer Nature 2018   357
A. E. M. Eltorai et al. (eds.), *Essential Orthopedic Review*,
https://doi.org/10.1007/978-3-319-78387-1_159

(continued)

Why are NSAIDs effective in treatment?	Cyclooxygenases and prostaglandin E2 is elevated by this benign bone mass. NSAIDs will reduce these levels
What are characteristic findings ofradiographs?	Cortical radiolucent nidus <1.5 cm surrounded by reactive bone
What is needed to make diagnosis of an osteoid osteoma?	Plain radiographs are typically diagnostic with biopsy rarely needed to confirm
What is the most common benign bone tumor?	Osteochondroma
What disease is the most common benign bone tumor associated with?	Multiple hereditary exostosis (MHE)
What is the gene of mutation and inheritance pattern?	EXT1. Autosomal dominant with variable penetrance. Affect the prehypertrophic chondrocytes of the physis
What is the treatment for MHE?	While surgery for resection is an indication if lesions are large enough to cause symptoms, many patients can be followed-up with observation alone. Most patients are asymptomatic and never seek medical attention at all
Where are giant cell tumors typically found?	Metaphysis of long bones in middle age (30–50) females
How do they appear on radiographs?	Eccentric lytic lesions

Chapter 160
Malignant Bone Tumors

Adam Driesman, Jose M. Ramirez, and Richard Terek

What patient demographic is most commonly affected by osteosarcoma?	Young adults. Mostly occur in the second decade of life during adolescent growth spurt
What skeletal sites are most common for osteosarcoma?	Areas of rapid bone turnover. Distal femur, proximal tibia, proximal humerus

(continued)

A. Driesman, MD (✉)
Department of Orthopaedics, NYU Langone Orthopedic Hospital, New York, NY, USA

Drs. Ramirez and Terek are at associated with Brown University, Providence, RI, USA
e-mail: adam_driesman@brown.edu

J. M. Ramirez, MD
Department of Orthopaedic Surgery, Alpert Medical School of Brown University, Providence, RI, USA

R. Terek, MD
Warren Alpert Medical School of Brown University, Providence, RI, USA
e-mail: richard_terek@brown.edu

© Springer International Publishing AG, part of Springer Nature 2018   359
A. E. M. Eltorai et al. (eds.), *Essential Orthopedic Review*,
https://doi.org/10.1007/978-3-319-78387-1_160

(continued)

How can osteosarcomas be subcategorized	Primary (85%) vs. secondary Surface subtypes: Perosteal, periosteal, high grade surface Intramedullary subtypes: Conventional, telangiectatic, low-grade, small-cell
What symptoms are associated with osteosarcomas?	New-onset pain over several months, swelling, fever. Pain may disrupt sleep
What is the most important prognostic factor at time of diagnosis?	Tumor stage Other poor prognostic factor in response to chemotherapy
What is typically seen on imaging for an osteosarcoma?	Classically periosteal reaction (Codman's triangle). Lesion with ill-defined borders, osteoblastic and/or osteolytic features
What is the treatment for osteosarcoma?	Limb salvage/wide resection + preoperative and postoperative multi-agent chemo
What are survival rates for osteosarcoma?	Survival rates surpass 70%
What age range are chondrosarcomas typically found in?	40–60 for primary lesions 25–45 for secondary: Arises from preexisting benign cartilage lesions (i.e., multiple enchondromas and multiple hereditary exostosis
In what locations are chondrosarcomas typically found?	Pelvis, proximal femur, proximal humerus
What genetic translocation results in Ewing sarcoma?	t(11:22). Formation of fusion protein (EWS-FLI1)
What population is Ewing sarcoma the most common nonhematologic primary malignancy of bone?	Patients younger than the age of 10

Chapter 161
Myositis

Stuart T. Schwartz

What is a **heliotrope rash**?	A lilac colored periorbital rash seen in dermatomyositis
What are "**mechanic's hands**"?	Cracked and fissured skin on the fingers of patients with dermatomyositis
What antibodies are present in myositis patients associated with interstitial lung disease?	**Anti-synthetase antibodies**
What serious underlying condition needs to be looked for in patients diagnosed with polymyositis and dermatomyositis?	Underlying malignancy

(continued)

S. T. Schwartz, MD
Alpert Medical School of Brown University, Providence, RI, USA
e-mail: sschwartz@lifespan.org

© Springer International Publishing AG, part of Springer Nature 2018   361
A. E. M. Eltorai et al. (eds.), *Essential Orthopedic Review*,
https://doi.org/10.1007/978-3-319-78387-1_161

(continued)

What blood test is typically elevated in inflammatory myopathy?	CPK
What myositis-specific antibody is seen with dermatomyositis skin rash?	**Anti-Mi-2**
What are **Gottron's plaques?**	Erythematous to purple lesions, present over the IP and MCP joints in patients with dermatomyositis

Index

© Springer International Publishing AG, part of Springer Nature 2018   363
A. E. M. Eltorai et al. (eds.), *Essential Orthopedic Review*,
https://doi.org/10.1007/978-3-319-78387-1